Radiating Knowledge

The Story of The Middlesex Hospital
Schools of Radiography

Edited by Adrienne Finch

disco

First published in the United Kingdom
by disco in 2012

Disco is the publishing arm of 'The Middlesex Hospital School of Radiography History Trust'. It has been accepted by HMRC as having charitable status with the following HMRC number XT27670. All profits from the sale of this book will go to radiographic charities.

© disco 2012
ISBN: 978-0-9571625-0-1

British Library Cataloguing in Publication Data
A catalogue record for this book is available from the British Library.

Printed in the UK by Halstan Printing Group, Buckinghamshire

Edited by Adrienne Finch
Design and layout by Jane Twydle

*To Marion Frank and
Mary Craig who inspired us all.*

CONTRIBUTORS

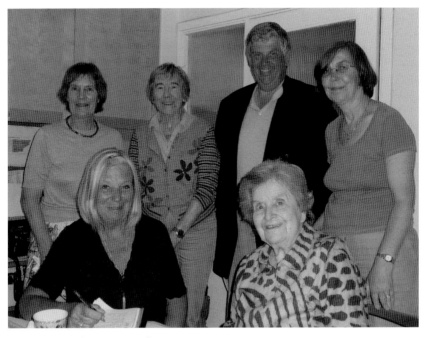

Image 1: A working party meeting

Back Row: Patricia Ducker, Adrienne Finch, John Twydle, Mary Embleton
Front Row: Sue Boult, Marion Frank

Adrienne Finch

Middlesex Hospital 1957-1961 (Student & Radiographer); 1964-1966 (Senior Radiographer & Assistant Tutor); 1975-1981 (Tutor & Deputy Principal); 1991-1997 (Principal Lecturer, University of Hertfordshire); College of Radiographers, National Coordinator clinical assessment scheme; 1998 Silver Medal of the Society and College of Radiographers: 1992-2005 ISRRT Director of Education (Europe & Africa).

Mary Embleton

Middlesex Hospital 1969-1971 (Student); 1977-1979 (Student Teacher); 1980-1990 (Principal, School of Radiotherapy); 1996-2008 Professional Officer at the Society and College of Radiographers; 1995 MA in Higher and Professional Education.

John Twydle

Middlesex Hospital 1972-1974 (Student); 1976 Medical Research Council at Northwick Park Hospital; 1978-1981 Middlesex Hospital, (Superintendent in Charge of CT scanner); Currently Customer Care Leader, Europe for GE Measurement and Control; 2009 Elected Fellow of the British Institute of Radiology.

Margaret McClellan

Middlesex Hospital 1975-1978 (Student Teacher & Deputy Principal); 1981-1990 (Co-ordinating Principal); 1984-1990 Member of Council of the Society of Radiographers; 1988-1990 Chair of Education and Training Committee; 1996-2000 Elected member of the Radiographers' Board of the Council Supplementary to Medicine; 1988-2006 Trustee of the Benevolent Fund of the Society of Radiographers; 2004-2006 Chair of the Trustees of the Benevolent Fund.

Stephanie Williamson

Middlesex Hospital 1980-1984 (Student and Radiographer); founder member of The Middlesex Hospital radio; founder of the Society of Radiographers Special Interest Group for Independent Practitioners; authored their professional standards; 2004-present, Head of Design and Health Care Planning at the Royal National Orthopaedic Hospital.

Christine Soutter

Middlesex Hospital 1958-1962 (Student diagnosis and therapy, and Diagnostic Radiographer); 1966-1969 (Senior/Superintendent Radiographer in Radiotherapy Department and School); 1969-1998 Superintendent Radiographer, Radiotherapy Department. Christie Hospital and Holt Radium Institute; 1977-1986 Council Member, College and Society of Radiographers; 1982-1983 President; 1998 Silver Medal of the Society and College of Radiographers; 1983-2005 Society of Radiographers Benevolent Fund Trustee: 2001-2004 Chair of the Trustees of the Benevolent Fund.

Nicholas Cambridge

Middlesex Hospital 1971-1977 (Medical Student); 1978 (House Surgeon); 1979 (Senior House Officer, Elderly Care); 1979-80, (Senior House Officer, Accident and Emergency); 1980-82, Registrar Radiology; 1982-84, Trainee GP, Barnet, Herts; 1984-2008, General Practitioner, Croydon; 2002, MD, University of London; 2007-present, Research Associate, Wellcome Trust Centre for the History of Medicine at UCL.

Ann Paris

Middlesex Hospital 1963-1969 (Assistant Tutor, Superintendent Radiographer); 1963 Archibald Reid Medal of the Society of Radiographers; 1969-1997 Radiology Services Manager, Northwick Park Hospital & Clinical Research Centre; 1977 Diploma of Medical Ultrasound; 1993-present, World Radiography Education Trust Fund, Trustee and/or officer.

CONTENTS

Contributors   4

Contents   7

Illustrations   9

Acknowledgements   17

Preface
by Professor Roger Berry   19

Foreword
by Sir Alan Langlands   20

Introduction
by Adrienne Finch   23

Chapter 1
Setting the Scene and the Hospital at War   26

Chapter 2
Building a modern profession 1949 – 1979   55

Chapter 3
Technical Innovation 1895 – 1991   80

Chapter 4
Reaching Out   106

Chapter 5
Two characters who shaped The Middlesex Schools   125

Chapter 6

Memories   147

Chapter 7

The Merger and the End   169

Bibliography   188

Appendix A

Middlesex Schools of Radiography lists of subjects and time allocation 193

Subjects and time allocation from Society/College of Radiographers

syllabi   194

Appendix B

The Role of the Professional Body and Statutory Regulatory Body

and the qualifications they awarded or recognised   196

Appendix C

Countries from which students came to study at The Middlesex

Hospital   200

Appendix D

Principals and Directors of the Schools of Radiography   201

Appendix E

Middlesex staff/former students elected President of Society of

Radiographers   203

ILLUSTRATIONS

Front cover image: The Middlesex Hospital. *Artist Thomas Shepherd, engraved by J Rogers, 1829.*

Image 1: A working party meeting. *Nicholas Cambridge.*

Image 2: The Middlesex Hospital Schools of Radiography at Doran House. *Working party collection.*

Chapter 1. Setting the Scene and the Hospital at War

Image 3: The Middlesex Hospital Chapel. *Carole Rawlinson.*

Image 4: Wilhelm Conrad Roentgen, 1906.

Image 5: The martyr's plaque. *John Twydle.*

Image 6: The Middlesex Hospital Electric Department 1919. Note the canary. *Working party collection.*

Image 7: The Middlesex Hospital appeal. *UCHL Archives.*

Image 8: Sir Edward Meyerstein. *Working party collection.*

Image 9: Bust of Sir William Collins by Jacob Epstein. *Working party collection.*

Image 10: H.R.H. The Duchess of York having her hand x-rayed at the opening of the x-ray department in 1935. *Working party collection.*

Image 11: Hand x-ray of H.R.H. The Duchess of York. 1935. *Working party collection.*

Image 12: Dr Harold Graham Hodgson. *Working party collection.*

Image 13: Sister Mary Craig. *Working party collection.*

Image 14: An underground operating theatre at The Middlesex Hospital. *UCHL Archives.*

Image 15: Bomb damage (National Temperance Hospital, 1941). *UCHL Archives.*

Image 16: Swimming pool in John Astor House. *Carole Rawlinson.*

Image 17: Sister Stella De Grandi. *Marion Frank collection.*

Image 18: Dr Graham Whiteside. *UCLH Archive.*

Chapter 2. Building a Modern Profession 1949 – 1979

Image 19: Marion Frank. *Working party collection.*

Image 20: Radiotherapy logbook. *Christine Soutter.*

Image 21: Diagnostic logbook. *Christine Soutter.*

Image 22: Kodak Course 1956. *Working party collection.*

Image 23: William (Bill) Stripp. *Royal National Orthopaedic Hospital.*

Image 24: The blue blazer and the hospital badge. *Working party collection.*

Image 25: Marlborough Court, Lancaster Gate. *Working party collection.*

Image 26: Teacher's Diploma of the College of Radiographers. *Society and College of Radiographers.*

Image 27: Chest x-ray. *John Twydle.*

Image 28: Doran House - plan of the second floor. *John Twydle.*

Image 29: Reception area column: Back row: Anne Wells, Christine Gill, Adrienne Finch, Marion Frank, Mary Embleton, Front row: Julia Lovell, Margaret McClellan. *Working party collection.*

Image 30: All Souls' primary school's rooftop playground and the adjacent rooftop terrace of the Schools of Radiography. *Exemplar Properties.*

Image 31: Middlesex Mice Christmas party in the School. Frankfurter distribution by Marion Frank. *John Twydle.*

Image 32: A prize winning student with Marion Frank and Marjorie Marriott (Matron). *Marion Frank collection.*

Image 33: Mary Craig. *Society and College of Radiographers.*

Image 34: Proceedings of workshop on computerised tomography. *John Twydle.*

Image 35: Margaret McClellan. *Working party collection.*

Chapter 3. Technical Innovation 1895 – 1991

Image 36: Marconi Deep X-ray unit. *Working party collection.*

Image 37: Telecobalt unit. *Working party collection.*

Image 38: Radiologist review console CT 5005. *John Twydle.*

Image 39: Professor JE Roberts. *Working party collection.*

Image 40: A 1986 nuclear medicine scan using physiology to detect disease. *Mary Embleton.*

Image 41: An early ultrasound scan. *John Twydle.*

Image 42: An ultrasound examination. *Working party collection.*

Image 43: An early x-ray tube. *John Twydle.*

Image 44: A light beam diaphragm in use. *Working party collection.*

Image 45: Kodak M3 processor. *Working party collection.*

Image 46: A bilateral mammogram. *Flavio Massari, bigstockphoto.com*

Image 47: Uwe Busch (Deputy Director of the Roentgen Museum in Germany), Godfrey Hounsfield, Marion Frank. *Marion Frank collection.*

Image 48: Original lathe bed CT prototype. *Courtesy of EMI Group Archive Trust.*

Image 49: MRI scan. *John Twydle.*

Chapter 4. Reaching Out

Image 50: Sir Brian Windeyer. *UCLH Archive.*

Image 51: Post diploma students at May and Baker. *Working party collection.*

Image 52: Fourth floor roof terrace, tutors and post diploma students. *Marion Frank collection.*

Image 53: Tyrone Goh, President of the ISRRT 2002-2006. *Tyrone Goh.*

Image 54: Philip Akpan. *Marion Frank collection.*

Image 55: The cassette loading area in a Gambian hospital 2000. *Jean Harvey.*

Image 56: Drying films processed by hand in a Gambian hospital 2000. *Jean Harvey.*

Image 57: Socialising at an ISRRT workshop in Arusha, Tanzania. *Marion Frank collection.*

Image 58: Teaching at an ISRRT workshop, South Africa. *Adrienne Finch.*

Image 59: Christine Soutter, President of the Society and College of Radiographers1982/83. *Society and College of Radiographers.*

Image 60: Donald Graham (2nd left) with others on a Middlesex organised trip. *John Twydle.*

Image 61: Julia Henderson and Marion Frank. *Radiography News.*

Image 62: Richard Evans. *The Society and College of Radiographers.*

Image 63: Margaret Lobo, President of Soroptomist International, 2008. *Margaret Lobo.*

Chapter 5. Mary and Marion

Image 64: Mary Craig as President 1957/58. *Society and College of Radiographers.*

Image 65: Marion Frank, Mary Craig and Margaret Wells on the award of the OBE to Mary, 1972. *Craig family collection.*

Image 66: Marion Frank as President 1967/68. *Society and College of Radiographers.*

Image 67: Royal Northern Hospital Pathology Staff 1938, on the left Ellen and on the right Marion Frank. *Marion Frank collection.*

Image 68: Ellen, Marion and Jean Harvey outside Buckingham Palace, 1981. *Marion Frank collection.*

Image 69: Table tennis at a garden party at Ellen's home. *John Twydle.*

Image 70: Marion studying the working party papers, Heron Court, 2010. *Nicholas Cambridge.*

Chapter 6. Memories

Image 71: Cartoon of Marion Frank certified by Marion as a true representation. *Jacqueline Wright.*

Image 72: 1940s students. *Marion Frank collection.*

Image 73: Receipt for fees, 1958. *Patricia Ducker.*

Image 74: A student wearing a Sister Dora cap. *Marion Frank collection*

Image 75: Underground tunnels. *Carole Rawlinson.*

Image 76: Performing a chest x-ray. *Marion Frank collection.*

Image 77: The Radioactive Saucies. *Geri Briggs.*

Image 78: Christmas lunch, fourth floor. *Margaret McClellan.*

Image 79: Dr Graham Whiteside. *UCLH Archive.*

Image 80: Marlborough Court cabaret in the 1950s, June Penney (Legg) second from left. *Marion Frank collection.*

Image 81: Cabaret chorus line of students, staff, radiographers and physicists. *Working party collection.*

Image 82: Jean Harvey ready to party as a punk rocker. *John Twydle.*

Image 83: An appreciative audience at a cabaret. *Working party collection.*

Image 84: The Order of the Frankfurter. *Working Party collection.*

Image 85: Middlesex students enjoying their first conference in the early 1980s. *Margaret McClellan.*

Chapter 7. The Merger and the End

Image 86: The Middlesex Hospital by Albany Wiseman, 1981. *Albany Wiseman.*

Image 87: The 1985 prize giving: Mary Robinson, Jennifer Edie, Julia Lovell, Mary Embleton, Professor Roger Berry, Margaret McClellan, Mary Lovegrove, Barbara Turner. *Margaret McClellan collection.*

Image 88: Margaret McClellan. *John Twydle.*

Image 89: Prize giving 1981 with Dr Rob Buckman as guest speaker. *Margaret McClellan collection.*

Image 90: The 1981 prize giving: the qualifying students with Dr Rob Buckman. *Margaret McClellan collection.*

Image 91: A lunch party to celebrate 50 years of radiography education at The Middlesex Hospital. *John Twydle.*

Image 92: The 50th anniversary lunch. *John Twydle.*

Image 93: Olive Deaville, President, with Margaret McClellan and Marion Frank. *Margaret McClellan collection.*

Image 94: The Christmas lunch, December 1980. *Working party collection.*

Image 95: Overhead view of The Middlesex Hospital's cleared site showing the Hospital Chapel and the Meyerstein façade still standing. *Exemplar Properties.*

End Page

Image 96: The Middlesex Hospital building site, showing the chapel and the Meyerstein façade still standing. *Exemplar Properties.*

Finally, although we have made every effort to trace copyright holders of images, due to the length of time since they were acquired we may inadvertently have omitted some people, and to those we apologise profusely. We will rectify these omissions in any subsequent edition.

ACKNOWLEDGEMENTS

An enormous thank you to Annie Lindsay, archivist to University College London Hospitals (UCLH), who gave us access to records which we thought were buried and who answered many questions, some of them several times; to the Society and College of Radiographers who allowed us access to their records; to Christine Hodgson whose professional editorial help, firm encouragement and expertise were invaluable; to Jane Twydle for the design and layout and for expert advice; to Marion Frank, the inspiration and initiator of the work; to Julia Merrick who initially made us believe we could actually write the book, and to all members of the working party: Adrienne Finch; John Twydle; Mary Embleton; Sue Boult; Patricia Ducker; Margaret Wells (to 2010); Nicholas Cambridge (from 2010), Stephanie Williamson (from 2011); to Margaret McClellan, Christine Soutter, corresponding members; to Anita Patel and Julia Solarno, current members of staff at UCLH who provided legitimacy to our status as part of the trustee funds of UCLH, to Nicola Twydle for providing hospitality, super food and refreshments for our all-day editorial meetings.

We should like to acknowledge all those who have made the time and effort to contribute their memories, some written and some recorded, many of them very busy people: Geraldine Stuart (Stevenson), Graham Buckley, Jenny Davidson (Richmond), Mary Medhurst (Pluister), Jean Barlow, Theo Campbell (Gibbs), Chin Jin Hon, Tyrone Goh, Jemeliah Rouse, Margaret Lobo, Olive Deaville, Susanne Forrest (Fairbrother), Jennifer Edie, Richard Evans, Marilyn Swann (Walton), Jean Harvey, R.P.Bhatnager, Barbara Turner (Allen), Marjorie Moyle, Anne Mackereth (Winterton), Sue Boult (Wilshire), Anne Ashmore (Wells), Diane Bennett and the many past international students at The Middlesex Schools of Radiography who answered our questionnaire.

The authors have relied heavily on the National Archives web site for currency conversions (http://www.nationalarchives.gov.uk/currency/). The 2005 figures are the latest available and are given in brackets after the sum mentioned.

We would also like to thank those who gave their permission to reproduce photographs, who include: Marion Frank's family who provided a number of pictures from her private collection; Mary Craig's family; Carole Rawlinson for the use of three reproductions of photographs from her book *Middlesex Memories*, the Hospital Chapel, the underground tunnel and the swimming pool; the Society and College of Radiographers for the pictures of Marion Frank and Mary Craig used in Chapter 5; the Royal National Orthopaedic Hospital for the picture of Bill Stripp; Albany Wiseman for the picture of the Middlesex Hospital in 1981; Uwe Busch for the photograph of him with Marion Frank and Godfrey Hounsfield; EMI Group Archive Trust for the photograph of the original lathe bed CT prototype and last of all, Exemplar Properties for the photographs of the cleared site that was The Middlesex Hospital.

PREFACE

by Professor Roger Berry

The role of the radiographer has grown in importance and complexity almost continuously since Wilhelm Conrad Roentgen produced the first radiograph of his wife's hand. In the early days of x-ray imaging, the radiographer was expected to be able to make the x-ray machine, a potentially lethal piece of machinery, work as well as being able to produce images of suitable diagnostic quality. As the scope of medical imaging increased, so did the role of the radiographer. Paralleling the role of the radiographer in medical imaging, the complexity of radiotherapy in the management of malignant disease required new and broader training for therapy radiographers, and visionary pioneers established schools of radiography to meet these new challenges. I am proud to have been so closely associated with The Middlesex Hospital Schools of Radiography and Radiotherapy during my years as the Sir Brian Windeyer Professor of Oncology at The Middlesex and as Chairman of the Education Committee, and to have been asked to contribute a short preface to this historic volume. The Schools have been recognised as being in the forefront of training radiographers for their entire lifetime, with the emphases changing as the needs of the profession have changed. The Staff deserve great credit for recognising early on that the provision of high quality medical imaging and treatment was a need reflected not just in highly developed countries, but also in the Third World, and their involvement in training radiographers from the Commonwealth and overseas is second to none. The quality of the science which they have taught has been equalled by their emphasis on the human side of their task, remembering always that at the centre of their role is a frightened patient. I hope that you enjoy reading this history of the work of some truly amazing people.

This book would never have been completed without the Herculean efforts over several years of the editor, Adrienne Finch, and the many contributions of John Twydle, labouring quietly in the background. They deserve our profound thanks.

FOREWORD

by Sir Alan Langlands

I can pinpoint my strongest memory of the Schools of Radiography and Radiotherapy at The Middlesex with chilling accuracy to 17 December 1983. The 'Middlesex Mice' Christmas party – an annual event for the children of hospital staff. It was, as usual, being hosted by the schools – it was in full swing when just after 1.30 pm it was interrupted by a cacophony of telephones and 'bleeps'. Not for the first time the hospital was being asked to respond to a bomb blast in London, on this occasion the Harrods' bomb which is believed to have killed four police officers and injured 90 people. There was no shortage of medical staff or on call radiographers that day and a hospital community that always knew how to enjoy itself quickly changed tack and went to work with calm professionalism, expertly caring for the wounded and distressed.

This book captures the essence and the spirit of The Middlesex Schools of Radiography and Radiotherapy, renowned for the education and professional development of radiographers but also contributing to high standards of service and ground-breaking research and an ethos which was second to none.

These strengths helped shape and inform a realignment of professional education and the merger of The Middlesex into University College London Hospitals, now home to one of the best equipped centres in the UK for diagnosing and treating injury and disease. The Hospital remains at the forefront of imaging diagnosis and the treatment of cancer. Interventional radiology, ultrasound, vascular and endovascular services, computed tomography, magnetic resonance imaging, digital plain film, fluoroscopy and nuclear medicine are all supported by cutting edge digital picture archiving and advanced communications. A new Cancer Centre was opened in April 2012. Highly technical treatment modalities with state of the art equipment, incorporating sophisticated imaging of their own, are able to accurately target tumours and spare normal tissue. The department also has a large molecular radiotherapy workload, which it collaborates with Nuclear Medicine to deliver. Radiographers deliver and continue to develop these pathways and modalities and as always the education is aimed at producing these highly skilled professionals. Of course, technological developments on this scale are not the result of spontaneous combustion – they have a proud history with deep roots in education and research.

The Middlesex Hospital and its Schools were very special. It is no coincidence that their historic coat of arms carried the inscription 'Miseris Succurrere Disco'. This comes from Virgil's Queen Dido aiding a shipwreck: 'Non ignara mali, miseris succurrere disco' (Not unacquainted with misfortune myself, I learn to succour the distressed). The Middlesex community did just that on 17 December 1983 and throughout its proud history, and this spirit lives on.

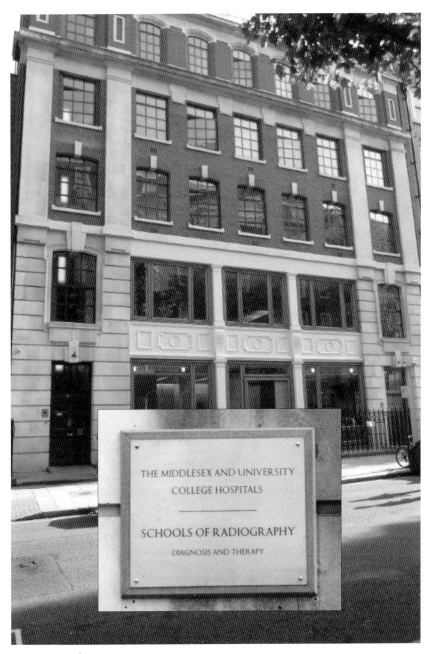

Image 2: The Middlesex Hospital Schools of Radiography at Doran House

INTRODUCTION

by Adrienne Finch

The original aim of this project was to gather and place in the archives of the University College London Hospital (UCLH), all appropriate material and records related to the history of the growth and development of the Schools of Radiography and Radiotherapy that could be found, in order to show how they adapted to meet the growing needs of patients and the community. We wanted to record for this and future generations the history of the education of radiographers at The Middlesex Hospital from 1935 to 1991, at which date all hospital based vocational schools were closed with contracts for education being placed with competing universities. The Middlesex School was amongst the first to be founded, and perhaps at the time it was typical of others. The declaration of war on September 3, 1939 caused a hiatus in radiography education development, but after 1945 the School went on from strength to strength, gaining an ethos and a spirit second to none: its reputation became world wide. After six years of research, collecting written and verbal memories from former staff and students, the working party decided that rather than merely place what had been found in the archives, a book should be published.

The drive to do the work was originally inspired by Marion Frank, for many years the Principal of the School of Diagnostic Radiography and the Superintendent of the X-ray Department at The Middlesex Hospital. She it was who persuaded us all in her own unique way, usually via early morning phone calls, to form a working party and start the research. She sadly died before her inspiration came to fruition.

In 1935 diagnostic radiography was based wholly on the use of x-rays, on basic photographic technology and wet processing. Radiotherapy was based wholly on the use of x and gamma radiation to treat cancer and some other diseases with its concomitant deleterious effects on the patient, and, in the early days, on the staff. Patient care was given a strong emphasis. The resolve to minimise the use of ionising radiation in both diagnosis and radiotherapy not only gave rise to legislation to protect staff and patients but also to the foundation of professional societies who set standards of education and practice. The continued drive to develop and make more efficacious diagnosis and treatment is now leading to the speedy disappearance of the world of conventional radiography and radiotherapy. In 2012, diagnosis is based less and less on ionising radiation, and more and more on ultrasound and magnetic resonance imaging. Additionally, investigations of patient illness are carried out by other scientists based on pathology, chemistry and genetics. Digital imaging has almost entirely replaced x-ray film and wet processing. Treatment of cancer is now performed by a wide variety of scientists, and includes the use of the cyber knife and rapid arc technology and perhaps in the future, gene therapy. The world of the radiographer may well disappear within a relatively short time. The unforgiving closure of hospital-based vocational schools in the early 1990s led to the disappearance of many of their records, and in addition it entirely changed the nature of the education. The authors of this work felt it was important to record the world of radiography as it was, the contributions made by those who worked to guide and develop the Schools, and the direct support given by the radiographic, medical, nursing, scientific and technical staff of the hospital.

The fragmented evidence is partly stored in the cold, dry and dusty archives in a basement in London's Euston Road and partly in the memories of those who studied, taught and worked during that time. We have been fortunate to have been able to talk to some radiographers who trained in the 1930s and 40s as well as in more recent decades. But those who remember the early days are a small and elderly population which is ever diminishing and becoming increasingly fragile and forgetful. Some to whom we would have liked to talk are no longer here. Without interested individuals and this publication much of this history may never re-surface although hopefully it will never be destroyed.

The School of Radiography at The Middlesex Hospital on Mortimer Street, London was founded in 1935 as part of the rebuilding programme of the hospital and its x-ray and radiotherapy departments. The School, later to become Schools (separate examinations for diagnosis and therapy were only initiated in 1951), and the hospital developed into world-renowned centres of excellence, particularly in education, before both their closures. The Schools were closed in 1991 and the education was transferred, along with that of all the other schools in the North East

24

Thames Health Region, to London's City University. The hospital itself closed in December 2005, its staff and services being transferred to University College London Hospital. We hope to show how throughout their existence, the Schools at The Middlesex endeavoured to meet the educational and clinical needs of UK and Commonwealth radiographers world wide and how the Schools adapted to meet the changes not only in imaging and treatment but also in education.

There is one qualification which must be made. This book sets out to be the history of The Middlesex Hospital Schools. However, up to 1965 the X-ray and Radiotherapy clinical departments and the Schools were inextricably entwined. There were no separate budgets, little physical difference, and the staff were appointed both to the departments and as tutors to the School. The Chief Radiologist and Radiotherapist were the Directors of the Schools, and the Superintendents of the Departments and the Principals of the Schools were joint appointments. Thus much of the early history is about both department and school.

We have been working for six years; the errors and omissions are largely ours, partly because we have had to work with the material available to us. Where possible we have found the full names of the staff who are mentioned, but in some cases it has proved impossible. However, there is some material that we know existed but which is now missing. We have also worked with people whose memories are subjective. This is history.

Adrienne Finch.

CHAPTER 1

Setting the Scene and the Hospital at War

The Middlesex Hospital was established in 1745, much later than London's oldest hospitals, St Bartholomew's and St Thomas', which originated as religious foundations in the twelfth century. St Bartholomew's was built in the City of London in 1123 for 'poor diseased persons until they get work'. Shortly afterwards, on the south side of the river, a convent was founded which included among its activities 'the care of the sick' and this became St Thomas' Hospital. In the thirteenth century the Bethlem hospital was founded for the care of people with mental illness. These hospitals were the only medical provision apart from religious foundations, although you could seek treatment from physicians (providing you could pay their fees), surgeons, apothecaries or quacks. As the population of London started to expand there was a desperate need for more hospitals, and during the eighteenth century, which was a time of philanthropy, The Middlesex was one of five voluntary London hospitals set up, together with Westminster (1720), Guy's (1733), St George's (1733) and The London (1740). There were also the Lock Hospital, which opened in 1747, and which catered for those with venereal disease, and four lying-in hospitals, caring for pregnant women, including Queen Charlotte's, founded in 1739.

The Middlesex Hospital started as two small houses in Windmill Street, off the Tottenham Court Road. The houses were leased from a local landowner, a Mr Goodge, and the rent was £30 per year. There were eighteen beds (three of these were for accident cases) and the hospital looked after the 'sick and lame' of Soho and the slums of Seven Dials around St Giles-in-the-Fields. In 1747, The Middlesex became the first hospital in England limiting its maternity beds to married women. However, as the demand for these beds increased it became necessary to enlarge the hospital. The Windmill Street site could not be further developed and the matron had reported that it 'was undesirable that there should be two in a bed as sometimes found necessary'. The hospital therefore moved to a site in Marylebone Fields on Tottenham Court Road on the estate of Mr Charles Berners. Tottenham Court Road, which eventually became Mortimer

Street, was a very wet marshy area covered in ponds. A lease was signed for 999 years at £15 per annum. By 1757 the hospital had increased to 64 beds and more were added by building a west wing in 1766 and an east wing in 1780. The hospital's financial fortunes went up and down, with the rations of the nurses and servants frequently being cut, until in 1791, an anonymous donor, who turned out to be Samuel Whitbread, the brewer, gave it financial stability. A ward was established in his name, for the reception of persons afflicted with cancer, where they could remain 'till relieved by art or released by death'. It was then, in 1791, that the hospital began its special study of the treatment of cancer. Right up to its demolition, The Middlesex had a ward named in Whitbread's memory.

In 1767 The Middlesex Hospital was the first London Hospital to purchase an electrostatic machine to treat patients using a technique called Franklinism (the treatment of disease using electricity) developed by Benjamin Franklin. Later in 1794 a Report in the *Transactions of the Royal Humane Society* records that a young girl called Sophia Greenhill was brought to The Middlesex Hospital after falling from a window and being declared dead by the surgeons. Electric shocks from an electrostatic machine were applied to her chest and she was restored to complete health.

In 1785 the first London medical school had been opened at The London Hospital, later to become the Royal London. In 1836, The Middlesex opened a medical school for teaching medical students, only male students being admitted. Gradually The Middlesex added many other amenities and increased the number of beds to 295. They also added a new outpatients' department, a nurses' institute, and a laundry. There were many enlargements to existing buildings which allowed other special departments to be opened for medical electricity, and for ear, nose, eye, and throat diseases. Later, in 1874, the first anaesthetist was appointed to the medical staff.

In 1890 a beautiful Chapel was built and this, together with the Meyerstein Institute façade, is all that remains of the main buildings today following the demolition of the hospital a few years ago in preparation for a housing development. A plaque commemorating a Middlesex x-ray martyr can be seen inside the chapel.

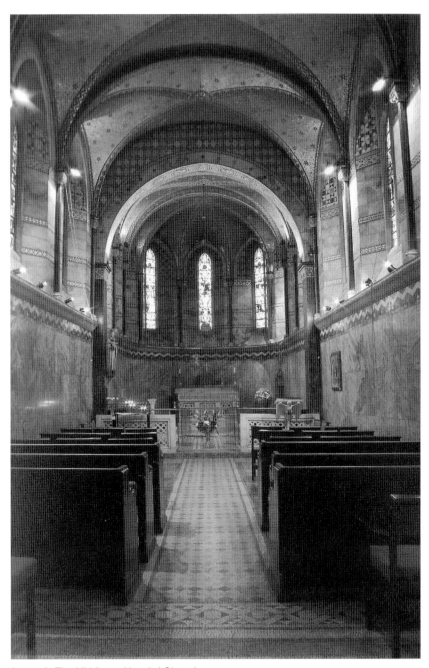

Image 3: The Middlesex Hospital Chapel

On 8 November 1895 Wilhelm Conrad Roentgen discovered x-rays in his laboratory in Wurzburg in Bavaria. He published only three papers on the topic, none of which included any of his own radiographs. He gave the first lecture on his discovery on 28 December 1895. On 1 January 1896 Roentgen wrote to scientific colleagues in several countries, including Lord Kelvin in Glasgow and Sir Arthur Schuster at the University of Manchester, enclosing some sample radiographs. Only the Schuster set survives and is preserved at the Wellcome Library, London. There was an article published about Roentgen's findings in the journal *Nature* in London on

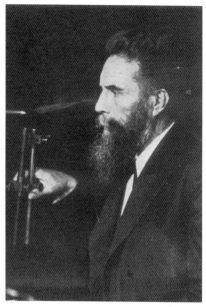

Image 4: Wilhelm Conrad Roentgen, 1906

23 January 1896. He never patented his discovery as he felt that the use of x-rays should be freely available for the benefit of society. He died in 1923, not of a radiation-induced condition.

Very shortly after this discovery The Middlesex Hospital acquired its first x-ray machine. Assembled at a cost of £14 (about £1000 today), it was installed in a small room over Casualty, which also housed the Hospital Administrator – whose duties were extended to include operating the x-ray set when required! The health risks of using x-rays were not immediately recognised although interestingly Roentgen himself did use lead shields and warned his visitors of the problems. As a result of this lack of knowledge, many people died as a result of the effects of radiation and were referred to as 'X-ray martyrs'. Causes of death included leukaemia and carcinoma of the skin, lung and pancreas.

The first Middlesex martyr was Reginald Mann, who joined the staff of the Electrical Department in 1899 as a radiographer. By 1906 he had had the first of many operations for cancers on his hands but up to three months before his death in 1916, at the age of 35, he operated the x-ray unit at The Middlesex Hospital convalescent home at Clacton, taking 'skiagrams', a term once used to describe radiographs of wounded soldiers. X-rays were also being used for treatment, following the 'like-for-like' philosophy that if it produced dermatitis it could also cure it. The long exposures required led to some consciousness of radiation protection, and by the time of the World War I *Knox's Textbook 4* contained the following warning:

> *The action of x-rays on tissues has been too well demonstrated by the unfortunate effects upon many of the early workers. An agent so capable of harmful effects must necessarily be treated with a considerable amount of respect when used for therapeutic purposes ... The first care of all workers should be to ensure the complete protection of the operator and attendants in an x-ray department, and there can be no doubt that at present too little attention is paid in most electrical cliniques [clinics] in this country to the important question of x-ray protection.*

Despite these warnings, those working with x-radiation still died. Sir Richard Doll showed that the cause of death due to various forms of cancer in 339 pioneer radiologists was significantly higher than in the normal population: for example carcinoma of the skin (7.8 times higher), leukaemia (6.2 times higher), cancer of the

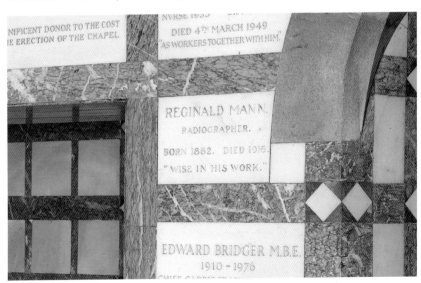

Image 5: The martyr's plaque

pancreas (3.2 times higher) and cancer of the lung (2.2 times higher). At The Middlesex a dedicated radiotherapy machine had been installed in 1904, although patients had earlier been treated using the same machines as those used for diagnosis.

The first director of the electrical department was Dr Cecil Lyster, who had been trained at Charing Cross Hospital and in 1902 joined The Middlesex, where he remained until his death from cumulative radiation injury in 1920. He had combined this appointment with a wartime role as medical officer to the electrical, massage and x-ray department at Queen Alexandra's Military Hospital, Millbank, next to Tate Britain. This hospital closed on 2 April 1977.

By 1923 the old hospital buildings were starting to deteriorate, and in 1925 a nursing sister, who was accompanying a patient on a trolley, had a lucky escape when a large mass of plaster fell from the ceiling just behind her. This acted as a stimulus for a critical survey by the architect and surveyor of the hospital which revealed that the general structure was unsafe in several places. The Board were presented with two alternatives: either to repair the structure at a cost of £10,000 (£300,000) or to rebuild. They decided on the latter. An appeal to the general public was started via a letter to *The Times*. The appeal, 'The Middlesex Hospital is falling down' was seen on hoardings, on buses, in papers and magazines throughout the country and in other parts of the world. The cost of rebuilding was born by donations alone, with

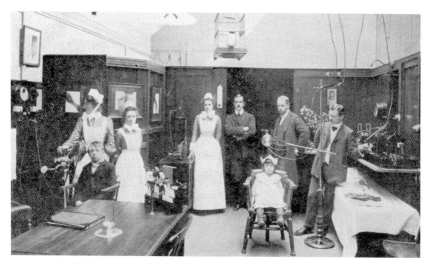

Image 6: The Middlesex Hospital Electric Department 1919. Note the canary

small donations coming from patients, staff, local traders and students, although there were many very large gifts from some rich and famous people.

Among the latter was Mr Edward Meyerstein, after whom the radiotherapy wing was subsequently named and whose story should be recorded especially. He was a London stockbroker, dealing on the South African gold market. In March 1934, he made a gift of £30,000 for necessary engineering works in order to open the east wing (which contained the x-ray department and the east wing wards). In July 1934 he gave a further £70,000 to complete the engineering and plumbing necessary for the east wing. In October, 1934, Mr Meyerstein, who was now a member of the Board of The Middlesex Hospital, asked permission of the Chairman (Prince Arthur of Connaught) to address the Board. He explained that this day was his birthday and he wished to give himself a present. The present he wished to give himself was the picture, then at the front of the hospital, which announced that a sum of £85,675 (£3,168,261.50) was still needed to complete the building of the hospital. He handed over a cheque for that sum to the Chairman and asked permission to take the picture! He also funded the purchase

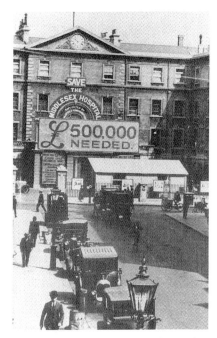

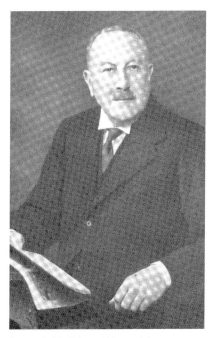

Image 7: The Middlesex Hospital appeal   *Image 8: Sir Edward Meyerstein*

of the athletics ground at Chislehurst with £10,000 and enabled the radiotherapy department to be built and equipped, initially donating £46,000. After ten years, in 1935, and at a cost of £1.25 million, the new hospital was opened by HRH The Duke of York, afterwards King George VI. Edward Meyerstein had donated a total of £242,000 (worth £9 million in 2005).

At a very early stage in the planning it had been decided that the department for diagnosis should be separate from that for treatment for the 'better advancement of both'. This was the first time this had been done. Most hospitals put the two departments together because they both used x-rays, not realising that they were fundamentally different. In 1933, a man who had previously made his money in industry, but whose life had been saved by the medical profession, became a substantial donor to medicine. Sir William H Collins made his first outstanding gift to The Middlesex, donating £50,000 for the building of the x-ray diagnostic department, 'the finest in the world', and then providing for its endowment with a gift of a further £50,000 (£1,850,000). Sir William Collins was Managing Director of the Cerebos Salt Company and was associated with Fortnum and Mason, Crosse and Blackwell and with Carreras. He had a deep admiration for the medical profession after his recovery from a serious illness which had necessitated his having three operations. The department was on the ground floor of the east wing. In September, 1933 the post of lead radiologist to the diagnostic x-ray department was offered to Dr Harold Graham Hodgson, who planned the department and made the decision to train radiography students.

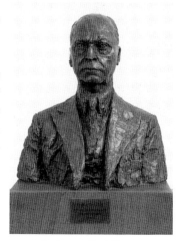

On May 29, 1935 the Collins x-ray diagnostic department was opened by the Duchess of York, who became the first 'patient', having her hand x-rayed. Such a procedure would not be allowed today, when each and every x-ray examination has to be justified by the benefit. A bust of WH Collins by Jacob Epstein took pride of place at the entrance to the department. Sir William Collins, who had been a Vice President of the hospital, died in December, 1947.

Image 9: Bust of Sir William Collins by Jacob Epstein

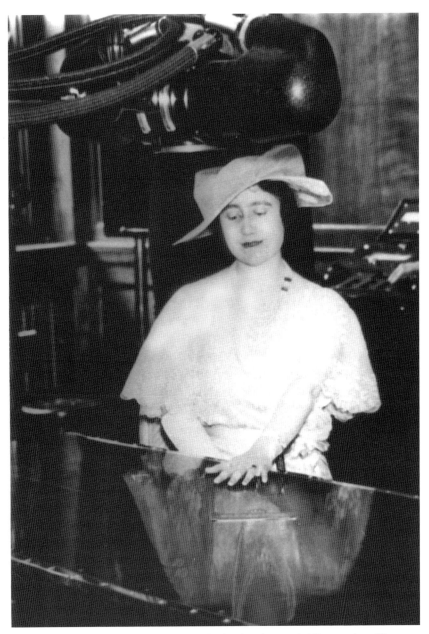

Image 10: H.R.H. The Duchess of York having her hand x-rayed at the opening of the x-ray department in 1935

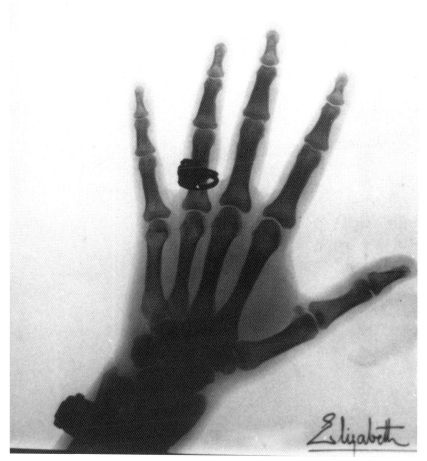

Image 11: Hand x-ray of H.R.H. The Duchess of York 1935

In the meantime, in the west wing, the radiotherapy department was built. Since 1930 The Middlesex had been providing consultant and expert support to the North Middlesex hospital in Edmonton, and the rapid growth of radiotherapy in the previous three years was acknowledged by the Chairman's report to the Board in 1933. Mr Edward Meyerstein had guaranteed £80,000 (nearly three million pounds). This substantial donation enabled radiotherapists to visit the principal radiotherapy centres in Europe in order that plans could be made to build and equip the best department possible. It was to have five floors, six out-patient treatment units, be adequately protected and capable of over six times the output and treatment then currently available. In May 1935 the contract was placed for the building at a cost of £18,000 (£666,000). On 1 January 1936 Dr Brian Windeyer was appointed to be in charge. However in March 1937 the opening of the radiotherapy department was deferred as Metropolitan Vickers, who were installing the equipment, had not completed their work. The Meyerstein Institute of Radiotherapy was finally, officially opened in 1938 by Sir William Bragg, President of the Royal Society, by which time Edward Meyerstein had been knighted.

Another substantial donor remained anonymous until well after the end of World War II. In June 1936 a lack of accommodation in the Nurses' home prevented an increase of staff. This anonymous benefactor donated £350,000 (nearly thirteen million pounds today) for an extension to the home with classrooms, recreation rooms and 105 bedrooms for sisters and nurses. It was stated that the donor's wish was to enable trainee nurses to have a collegiate life. It was not until well after the end of the war that the donor was found to have been JJ Astor, then Major Astor and Chairman of the Board, and subsequently to become Lord Astor. The home was named John Astor House.

However, it appears from the Board of Governors' minutes that although the capital had been obtained for the build there were continuing problems with paying the revenue bills. The income appeared to depend on donation, wealthy benefactors, income from private patients and bequests. 'The present grave financial situation of the hospital' is referred to in the November, 1935 Board of Governors' minutes. Negotiations for large overdrafts from the hospital's bankers continued right up to the outbreak of war. In February 1936 a small ward with twelve beds used for incurable cancer patients was to be closed, saving £1500 (£55,000) per annum, and to be re-opened for paying patients. In February 1937 the re-building fund itself was in deficit to the tune of £2,500 and by February 1938 there was an overdraft of £30,000 (£1.2 million) to the general fund, and £40,000 (£1.5 million) to the reconstruction fund agreed with the hospital's bankers. The fundraising had dealt with the rebuilding without real consideration for upkeep, maintenance and payment of staff and indeed these problems continued throughout the life of the hospital. Right up to the inception of the National Health Service, The Middlesex Hospital was funded by voluntary subscription.

The Society of Radiographers (encompassing both professional and union activities) was founded in 1920, when it was realised that standards had to be set in order to protect both staff and patients from the unwise and ill-educated use of ionising radiation. A syllabus was established with help from the Chartered Society of Massage and Medical Gymnasts (later to become the Chartered Society of Physiotherapy) founded in 1894 by four nurses. The first specialist radiography examination was held in February 1921 at the Royal College of Physicians' Examination Hall, Queen Square, London, a venue which continued to be used until the early 1980s. According to Michael Jordan, a former General Secretary of the Society, there was some criticism of the first examination, a tradition which continued unabated and with increasing enthusiasm over 75 years. By April 1923 the Council of the Society of Radiographers laid down regulations that a candidate for examinations should have received eight months' training as well as having performed twelve months' practical work in a department. The first inspection of schools took place in 1932 when four London schools were visited and officially recognised. These were Guy's, King's College Hospital, the Royal Northern Hospital and the Hospital of St John and St Elizabeth.

As has already been mentioned, the decision to train radiographers at The Middlesex was made by Dr Harold Graham Hodgson, director of the X-ray Diagnostic Department in 1934. By 1936 The Middlesex School was 'recognised' by the Society of Radiographers, together with the Royal and Western Infirmaries, Glasgow, St Vincent's Hospital, Dublin, the General Hospital, Johannesburg, and Melbourne Hospital, Australia in addition to the four previously mentioned. The qualification examination set by the Society of Radiographers was for both Diagnostic and Radiotherapy (separation of the two modalities not occurring until 1951). Dr Graham Hodgson and a fellow radiologist, Dr JH Graham Webster had drawn up a suggested prospectus and set out to recruit students (Appendix A). Dr Graham Hodgson proposed that the Sister in Charge of the Electrical School (Physiotherapy) should be tutor to the Radiography School as well. However, the organisation, staffing and costs of the proposed school did not appear to have been cleared with the House or Nursing Committees as a series of questions were posed to Dr Graham Hodgson, who had made a number of decisions without the Committees' authority. From the tone of the very carefully worded minutes this undoubtedly caused friction. He was also proposing to advertise for a resident radiography tutor without

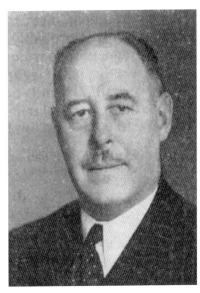

Image 12: Dr Harold Graham Hodgson

budget agreement. By February 1935 forty two application forms had been sent out, three students had actually entered and there was a possibility of a further seven, but no tutor had been appointed. Dr Graham Hodgson argued that his plans should be allowed, stating in a letter of 13 May 1935 that having a School of Radiography would save the hospital much expense. The radiography students would carry out about two thirds of the work in the department, saving the employment of additional radiographers. This tradition of using students as part of the workforce continued throughout the country for many years. Nowadays the functioning of a department must not be dependent on students and the number of students allocated to a clinical department is governed by having a sufficient number of radiographers to ensure adequate supervision and the amount and range of clinical work available. Dr Graham Hodgson also said that the necessary lectures would be given by himself and his assistants, and in equipment by Mr Morgan Davies, the consulting engineer to the x-ray department. Morgan Davies was still lecturing to the students in 1970, using exactly the same notes! Dr Graham Hodgson felt that these lecturers should receive a proportion of the students' fees. Mr Alfred Webb Johnson, a consultant, stated very firmly that radiography students should not be taught more about the apparatus and electricity than was within the knowledge of those in charge of the department.

The Nursing Committee resolved to advise the House Committee:

i.   It would be bad policy to endeavour to start the School with stop-gap arrangements.
ii. It saw no reason to depart from the usual practice of appointing a sister tutor to supplement lectures given by members of honorary staff.
iii. As Dr Graham Hodgson's assistants were already paid an honorarium for their services and their lectures were given in hospital time, there was no reason why they should be paid a proportion of the students' fees.
iv. The Committee recommended the retention of Mr Morgan Davies, as some of the apparatus in the newly designed x-ray department was unique, especially designed by him. Dr Graham Hodgson considered that his retention as lecturer to the students would prevent considerable expenditure on renewals and repairs due to errors in usage.
v.   The Committee considered that more use might be made of Sister Bristow [thought to be in charge of the electrical department].
vi. No appointment of a resident radiography tutor should be made until such time as the organisation of the departments of x-ray diagnosis, medical electricity and radiotherapy could be viewed as a whole.

It took some months of discussion before the situation was resolved. The Nursing and House Committees showed a preference for a nurse with a radiography qualification to be in charge of the students and the day to day organisation of the department. In the diagnostic department this continued until 1949, when Marion Frank, the first non nurse to hold the post, was appointed. Mary Craig, a qualified nurse, was designated to be superintendent of the radiotherapy department in 1942 and remained so until she retired in 1974. Initially staff nurses were appointed to both diagnostic and radiotherapy departments. The level of recruitment seemed to be very low at this time (1935) and the Hospital's national examination results were not satisfactory. The Society of Radiographers wrote to the hospital querying the failure rate, which appeared to be due to lack of knowledge in radiotherapy and it was felt that the students did not spend enough time in that department. In September 1936 the Lady Superintendent (Matron) reported that the Society of Radiographers had increased the period of training from one year to two, with the requirement that entrants should have the School Leaving Certificate, although this latter rule was rescinded barely eighteen months later. Dr Graham Hodgson recommended that the intake should be six students every six months and that each student should spend six months in the radiotherapy department.

The question of fees was also discussed in 1936, with £35 (£1,294) for the two year course being suggested. Contact was to be made with Guy's and King's College Hospitals to see if they would agree a similar fee. The Royal Northern was not mentioned, even though Kathleen Clark, who was to become the doyen of British radiography, was radiographer in charge there at that time. Miss Clark had sat the first qualification in 1921, having

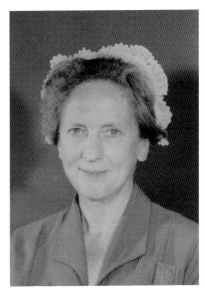

Image 13: Sister Mary Craig

gained her clinical experience at Guy's Hospital, and in 1935 she was the first woman that the Society of Radiographers elected as President, which was seen as a ground-breaking event. Two years later she wrote the book, *Positioning in Radiography*, which was the standard text for many years and whose thirteenth edition was published in 2005. However the texts were banned in some Middle Eastern countries because of the semi-naked women displayed for positioning purposes! This was a problem for ex-patriot radiographers working in the area who had no text to refer to in difficult cases.

At the end of September 1938 Neville Chamberlain signed the Munich agreement which allowed Germany to annexe the Sudetenland from Czechoslovakia, and it was noted in the Board of Governors' minutes of October 1938, that as part of the National Emergency Procedures The Middlesex Hospital was to be converted to a Casualty Clearing Station in the event of war. The actual emergency was over but a detailed plan was to be drawn up in case an emergency occurred again. It is clear that a further emergency was expected as planning then took place as follows. London and its outlying area of up to 60 miles out were to be divided into twelve sectors with a teaching hospital at the hub of each sector. Outside the centre there were to be two rings, with an advanced base and a base hospital. Dr Harold Boldero, Dean of the Medical School and officer in charge in case of war, presented a report to the Board on 16 March, 1939. He recommended:

> the purchase of 5,000 sandbags and a sandbag filling machine; blankets and wooden strips to gas proof the sub-basement and black paper for the windows; a supply of plywood to replace broken windows; blackout material; two units for fire fighting; splints and trestles for one hundred stretchers; an alternative telephone switchboard to be put in the basement; hoarding for the courtyard; a standby electrical generator; an increased stock of morphine and anti-gas gangrene serum. He also suggested that an estimate of the personnel required should be made for when the Hospital was converted to a 200 bed reception hospital.

In April 1939, an emergency meeting of the Nursing Committee was called. It was recommended and approved that all Schools, except for Nursing, should close for the time being and be re-opened when the situation allowed either in London or elsewhere. Students were advised to volunteer as mobile medical auxiliaries in the Middlesex sector. Assistants in the radiotherapy department were advised to revise their diagnostic training, presumably felt to be of more use in case of war. In June 1939 it was reported that the Central Emergency Committee was willing to meet the expenses of staff in the massage, electrical and radiography departments who volunteered for the examination in First Aid and Home Nursing. It was felt that this would give the students a better standing in the sector in the event of war. Action to be taken in the x-ray department in the case of an air raid warning included that all personnel should proceed to the department, and the radiographer was to ensure that all machines were switched off at the mains.

On 19 July 1939 the emergency war plans were accepted and it was agreed that if war were to be declared Dr Hugh Marriot would be appointed Medical Commandant. Key personnel were instructed not to go abroad during the summer recess.

On 29 August Emergency War Orders were promulgated. Some patients were to be evacuated and others moved to the third floor of the main building. Stretcher cases were sent to Reading. The outpatient department was closed and the annexe became a first aid post. All medical personnel were to move into the hospital and all students and residents not allocated for duty at the hospital were to vacate their rooms. Those allocated to sector hospitals were to proceed there, and if there was no sleeping space allocated, were to proceed to Town Halls for billeting. All persons on duty were to carry a respirator (in case of gas attack).

War was finally declared on 3 September 1939, although it had been expected for much of the previous year. By end of the month, the Ministry of Health (MoH), without making clear who was financially responsible (was it ever thus!), gave instructions that the hospital was to be cleared and 200 beds made available for casualties. The Hospital's income had dropped severely because donors thought that the Ministry was running the hospital. In the early days of the war routine work came to a standstill but 'normal service' had to be resumed because of the need to treat local patients. Pressure was put on the Ministry of Health to allow the outpatient department to be opened for the civilian sick. At the hospital, the Emergency War Committee was set up with fortnightly meetings and it was agreed that a Board meeting would now only be called as and when necessary. Dr Hugh Marriot, the Medical Superintendent, wished to join the Royal Army Medical Corps (RAMC) and Dr Alan Moncrieff was appointed to fill the vacancy. This change of medical staff because of their volunteering for army service was to cause problems throughout the war. By the end of the year 120 beds were re-opened (the maximum allowed by the MoH).

Although the x-ray diagnostic and radiotherapy clinical departments had been founded and the decision to train students had been made and the first students had been taken on, a hiatus in the development of both clinical departments and education was caused by the war, as the needs of the country, the armed services, the hospital, and at times the need to survive, took precedence. All the junior students were sent home without ever having had a lecture. Eventually they were sent to Middlesex sector hospitals, which included Tyndall House, Aylesbury and Stoke Mandeville, although one student, Nan Harris, was forgotten and later contacted the hospital to ask what she should do. Geraldine Stuart (Stevenson), a student in 1939, mentioned that 'lectures were given in a very disorganised and ad hoc way, physics delivery was very hit and miss, with knowledge of radiography protection being acquired as radiographic technique was learnt, practically in the department'. There were odd lectures on photography at Tyndall House by

JM Kenny, who was more interested in identifying the enemy aircraft flying overhead than lecturing to the students, and Geraldine had one lecture on radiotherapy by Dr Brian Windeyer. There were recorded meetings of the Nursing Committee up to June 1940, but there was then a two-year gap to 1943, at which time the tone of the minutes, and the subjects discussed, made clear that defeat and invasion was now unlikely, although the war might continue for some time. Thus in November 1939, the radiography students evacuated to the outer sector at Aylesbury returned to London during the period of the 'Phoney War'. Details of lectures in physics were outlined, and the course fees to be paid were specified. The course had been reduced to 18 months and the fee reduced from £45 to £40. Qualification examinations were reasonably successful with there being only one failure out of eight entries.

Apart from the Emergency War Committee, other committees appeared not to meet, or not to meet very frequently, and records are sketchy.

On 28 September 1940, a bomb fell on the Annex, and it was decided that brickwork to the windows should now be continued to the top. All Souls' School, next door to the hospital, had been severely damaged. The number of patients was sixty three (normally two hundred), but one hundred and thirty air raid casualties had been admitted during the month. A bomb fell on the laundry at Hendon in November, and there was a large amount of glass damage to the

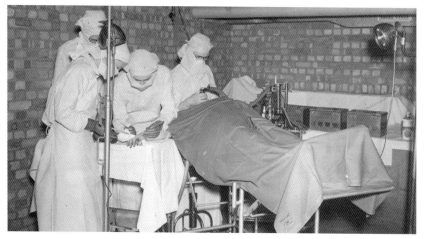

Image 14: An underground operating theatre at The Middlesex Hospital

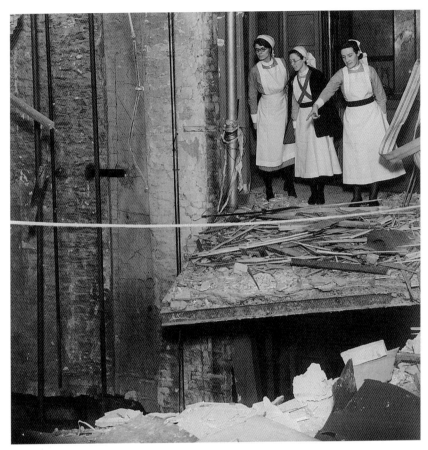

Image 15: Bomb damage (National Temperance Hospital, 1941)

front of the hospital. In December congratulations were sent to the staff on the reception of a large number of casualties. Despite the failure of the electrical supply, thirty incendiary bombs had been dealt with. On 31 January 1941 two 100lb high explosive bombs fell on the hospital, with one person killed and one student being severely injured. Twenty three air raid casualties were admitted on 8/9 March and eighty four casualties on 16 April. There followed a detailed report on the air raid of that night:

> *The surgical organisation was tested to the extreme, but the staff coped with twice the number of casualties than had previously been experienced. Operating did not finish until 24 hours later. The Boy Scouts were on the go*

the whole time. Nurses on duty were unflaggingly courteous. The person reporting wondered when they ate. Damage was inflicted on the 4th, 5th and 6th floors of the North East wing, and the North ward of the Annex.

It was resolved that all the ground floor windows were to be bricked up as the blackout curtaining was blown out so frequently, and by July all second floor wards were bricked up.. The cost of repairs and bricking up had to be negotiated with the War Damage Commission and cost £1396 9s (£40,106).

Throughout the remaining period of the war, at each meeting of the Emergency War Committee the number of patients in the hospital was reported alongside the number sent out to the sector, presumably to be out of reach of the London bombing. Numbers of patients varied from 98 to close to 200 with upwards of 95 being sent to the sector in each fortnightly period.

In April 1941, the committee requested the Ministry of Labour to define all hospital men and women employees as 'Essential War Workers'. There was a constant battle with engineering staff, cleaners, porters and ancillary workers being called up, and tragically some being killed at their homes. Keeping the level of staff required to function was difficult. The following month the hospital was registered as 'a protected industry'.

The Board met in May and it was found that income was greater than expenditure due to legacies, and it was agreed that some of the overdraft was to be paid off. An invasion practice was held. In September 1941 the number of civilian sick had increased and the number of beds occupied by them had exceeded the number authorised by the Ministry. In the following December twenty five cases of ringworm were treated. It was reported to the Board that there had been no further air raids since the previous Board meeting. The reopening of the outpatient annex was to be considered because of the increasing number of patients. By June 1943 the committee agreed to open forty additional beds for the civilian sick, but it was deemed unnecessary to inform the Ministry of Health.

In January 1943 there was a report of two air raid casualties admitted with four being seen in outpatients. A protocol was devised of actions to be taken during an alert. The Preliminary Training School (trainee nurses in their first three months) was to shelter in the department, the massage department was to be closed, and maternity patients were to be transferred to the first floor of the east wing. At the beginning of 1943, three senior sisters already past retirement age were to continue to work.

A paper on the future of the medical services indicated that it looked as though the 'freedom of medical practice would appear to be in jeopardy' - the first hint of the foundation of the National Health Service.

In May 1943, a penicillin research committee was established as there was to be a ward set aside for patients being treated with penicillin as part of research into its efficacy. Alexander Fleming had first noticed the effect of a mould on bacteria in 1928, but it was not until 1938 that Howard Florey and Ernst Chain, a German refugee working at Oxford University, isolated the bacteria-killing substance, penicillin, so that it could be produced as a drug. At first supplies were very limited and the patients at The Middlesex were part of the clinical trials. But an American drugs company started to mass produce it and by D Day in June 1944 sufficient was being produced to treat all the bacterial infections that broke out in the troops. The trials continued at The Middlesex from May 1943 onwards, despite the theft of some penicillin being reported. There is no record either of an investigation or a culprit being found.

The Board was obviously beginning to think of a post-war future and the expansion of the hospital, as they attempted to buy the freehold of some surrounding properties to enable the rebuilding of casualty and outpatients. Reconditioning of the latter would cost £5000 (£129,760) and in the event the Ministry of Health would not agree the expenditure. The rebuilding never took place. A seven-a-side rugby tournament was run by the medical students to raise funds for the hospital and £352 was raised (£1,950), but a request for a hospital dance was refused. Members of the allied forces were not permitted to attend dances in the nurses' home.

In December 1943, the whole of the third floor was opened for nurses and students ill with flu, and in March 1944 there was an outbreak of smallpox at Mount Vernon Hospital. This latter was of concern because Middlesex Hospital nurses and radiography students were assigned there.

Life for the radiography students must have been difficult as they were shuttled to and from the hospitals in the sector and The Middlesex depending on the severity of the bombing and the deemed risk of invasion. In January 1940, it had been decided to re-open the Medical School and the Preliminary Training School for nurses. But by September, when the bombing of London was becoming severe, senior radiography students were retained at the main hospital, the rest being dispersed to sector hospitals. Final examinations had been taken and passed by six students and qualification examinations continued to be held throughout the war. There was obviously still an issue with The Middlesex students' knowledge of radiotherapy practice as there were enquiries from the Society of Radiographers in January 1941 as to how much time they spent in radiotherapy. The following month meetings of the Nursing Committee were suspended, but they still had time to consider whether a radiography student who had married could be allowed to continue her training (she was!). In April 1941 it was stated that 'thefts from the Nurses' home' continued and the police were informed. A skeleton was purchased for the instruction of the radiography students, but at that time there was no allocated budget to buy books or teaching aids; these could only be obtained by special application. In June 1941 it was reported that the Ministry of Labour and National Service had agreed that it was not necessary for massage and radiography students to abandon their studies to take up war work but the School of Radiography was not allowed to accept foreign students as it could not be guaranteed that they would not come into contact with service personnel.

In June 1942 the pre-clinical medical students were to return from Leeds where they had been for the previous two years. Apparently the risk from air raids and the chance of invasion was felt to be low enough to allow this. In July the Emergency War Committee took time to resolve that radiography students should not be classified as university students by the Ministry of Labour. Even at this early stage the medical profession was concerned that radiographers and other ancillary professions should not be allowed the status of a university education. It was not until 1991, despite ongoing pressure throughout much of this time, that the radiography qualification finally attained degree status.

In December 1943, it was resolved that 'lady visitors' to medical students in residence be allowed between 2pm and 7pm, whilst for medical officers there was an extension to 10pm. In March 1944 the University of London resolved that

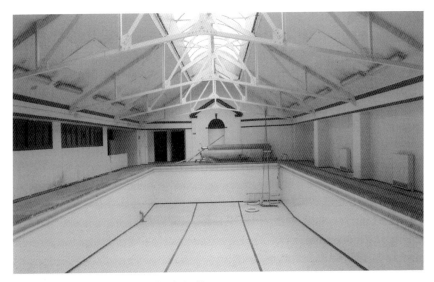

Image 16: Swimming pool in John Astor House

male and female students be treated equally. The Middlesex did not take female medical students at all until 1947.

Despite food and clothing rationing there were ongoing and quite severe shortages in basics, with items considered luxuries being completely unobtainable. By the end of 1939 even the water in the swimming pool was offered to the London Fire Brigade for an emergency supply. At the end of 1939 the butter ration was 4ozs (about 110 grams) per person per week. By February 1941 difficulties in the supply of food are mentioned and it was a stated aim to keep one week's supply of tinned food in the hospital. In January 1942 the hospital egg ration was reduced from 1,700 per week to 175, allowing one per week for gastric patients and one per month for all the other patients and the staff. Nurses were given permission to keep rabbits behind the nurses' home to help with special diets. The milk ration was reduced from seven pints per person per week to five. By September the milk ration had been reduced again to 384 pints per week for staff and patients – what this was per head is not known, but if there were 200 patients and a commensurate number of living-in staff the reduction must have been drastic. A donation of green vegetables was gratefully accepted and the use of dried eggs discussed at the Emergency War

Committee. In May 1943, 950lb of tinned poultry was bought at the cost of three shillings and sixpence per pound (£4.50p).

In December 1941 it was difficult to obtain curtain fabric for the scabies clinic. The soap ration of three ounces per month per person was deemed insufficient. In May the soap ration was increased and nurses were allowed to buy soap outside the hospital. In April 1943 a gift of 288 gross tubes of toothpaste was gratefully accepted. In February 1942, patients' notes from the years prior to 1912 were sent for re-cycling, and x-rays prior to 1934 were released as they were in great demand in the aircraft industry which processed and used the residual chemicals. Rover scouts had worked for three weeks sorting out the x-ray film of which two tons had raised £90 (£2,600). In June 1942, the headmaster of All Souls' School requested that the hospital coke stored in the school playground be moved. It was still in situ a year later with the alternative use of the bomb site of the German church being suggested, but this was deemed unsuitable because of the large amount of rubble. In March 1943 the railings of the convalescent home at Clacton had been requisitioned, for which £4 16s 7d (£139) was received as compensation.

In September 1943, it was discovered that a large quantity of linen had been stolen from the Nurses' home. The value of linen lost, at pre war prices was £708 (£20,000); a female cleaner had been convicted of theft. In October a linen audit was instituted for the whole hospital. The value of missing linen was then £379 4s (£10,000), with an additional sixty pillows being lost.

In January 1942 there was for the first time a report to the Emergency War Committee of a shortage of domestic staff, the number needed being down by thirty five maids and cleaners. This was monitored at every succeeding meeting but severe shortages continued to the end of the war. In May 1943 the company providing male cleaning staff were unable to recruit any staff and asked to be released from their contract. In June, equality of pay with men for a female porter was refused. A radiotherapy clerk was called up for work in industry and it was considered worthy of note that a 'creole' had been accepted for training. This term accurately means a person of mixed African and European descent, but here probably means a black person.

In 1939, it was agreed that radium treatments should continue to be carried out at the hospital's radiotherapy department rather than establish treatment centres outside London with the problems that protection and the training of staff would cause. In August 1940 Dr Margaret Snelling (later to become director of the radiotherapy department and school) was appointed to the radiotherapy department at a salary of £250 (£7,200) per annum. At the end of September, a period heralding the bombing of London, it was decided that radiotherapy would be continued 'for those considered to be worthwhile', but that Mount Vernon Hospital, in Northwood, Middlesex, be asked to treat Middlesex Hospital patients using Middlesex staff. The equipment was to be dismantled and stood down, with the exception of items necessary for the treatment of outpatients. This decision was bedevilled throughout the war by the very great difficulty of the two hospitals sorting out the finance and control. It was finally resolved, for in December, it was stated that observation windows for the treatment rooms were to be sent to Mount Vernon from The Middlesex Radiotherapy department, as the special protective glass could not be sourced elsewhere. In September 1941, the St Thomas' deep x-ray machine was out of action due to tube breakdown and an old Middlesex one was loaned at no cost. In July 1943 an application was made to the British Red Cross for the provision of an additional superficial x-ray treatment set. In July 1942, Dr Brian Windeyer was appointed a Professor of the University of London. He was receiving £400 (£11,500) per annum for being medical commandant.

In the middle of July 1940 emergency x-ray rooms were fitted out at a cost of £29 18s (£860) and in December a radiographer was appointed at a salary of £2 15s (£79) per week. In January 1941, replacement intensifying screens costing £19 7s 3d (£556) and an x-ray tube costing £78 (£2,250) were authorised. In April, four valves were replaced at a cost of £210 (£6,000). Under the 'Bundles for Britain' scheme two sets of Victor portable x-ray machines were donated. The 'Bundles for Britain' organisation was founded in early 1940 (before the USA's entry to the war) by Mrs Wales Latham, a New York socialite, to provide non-military aid to the British people. They collected items such as medicine, clothing and blankets from American citizens and shipped them to Britain. A Picker unit was purchased from the Red Cross. The firm Picker International was an American firm, which, during World War II was the only company producing mobile field x-ray units for the Allied Forces. (These were still in use in 1959, but were not popular as they were heavier and more unwieldy than Little Picker, also American and apocryphally said to have been later dropped at D Day!). On 25 June 1941 Sister R Smith was appointed to be in charge of both x-ray and radiotherapy, but by the end of the year the two roles were separated and Sister Joan Parbery designated in charge of x-ray at a salary of £130 plus £80 for living out (£6,000). In June 1942 there were staff difficulties in radiology where two members of staff had been found to have low blood counts; the staffing of the x-ray department in September, 1942 was two full-time and one part-time radiologist. In December

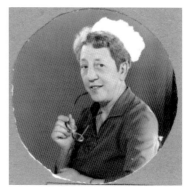

Image 17: Sister Stella De Grandi

Dr Graham Hodgson asked for the return of two rooms currently in use as a night casualty room and first aid post, and this was agreed as long as x-ray tubes and valves were available; it would cost £255 (£6,600). The tomography unit was to be returned to hospital from Tindall House at a cost of £20 (£574). Intensifying screens were replaced at a cost of £230 (£6,600).

In March 1943 the salary scale recommended by the Society of Radiographers was accepted with the bottom of the scale for senior radiographers being £250 per annum (£6,400). A decision was made that radiographers and masseuses should have pay equal to that of nurses but there was no extra for nurses with a supplementary certificate in, for example, radiography. On 15 September, Stella de Grandi qualified as a radiographer. Sister de Grandi as she subsequently became, remained as Sister-in-Charge and deputy to Marion Frank as Superintendent Radiographer, until her retirement in 1970. She was regarded as an institution and one of the legendary parties with a cabaret was held in her honour when she left.

Sadly, Board of Governors and Emergency War Committee Minutes are missing from April 1944 to April 1946. Thus we have no record of the hospital's reaction to the D day landings, the end of the war or the attitude of the Board toward the National Health Service or the preparations for its institution.

However, it was reported to the Nursing Committee in October 1944 that there had been complaints from parents of radiography students at Stoke Mandeville hospital concerning the lack of lectures. That same month a sub-committee for education which included radiography, was appointed by the Emergency War Committee as there appeared to be no chain of responsibility for the school. The sub-committee comprised the chair of the nursing committee, the Medical Commandant, Professor Windeyer, and the Lady Superintendent (Matron). It had the power to co-opt and one of their first actions was to co-opt Dr Graham Hodgson. Amongst the first actions of this sub-committee were the following:

i.   to define the number of lectures to be given as set out in a schedule.
ii. to resolve that radiography students should be brought back to The Middlesex from Tindall House and Stoke Mandeville, and that lectures to them should be given as per the schedule.
iii. that all lecturers should be appointed under the procedure set out by the Medical Committee.
iv. that nursing sisters in the school should undertake more teaching within their province and that assistance should be given to them to acquire teaching qualifications.

On 1 January 1946, the length of radiography training was restored to two years and the course content agreed (Appendix A). In June, Sister Lucy Mary Craig (radiotherapy) and Sister Joan Parbery (diagnostic) were appointed as Superintendent Radiographers and Tutors at a salary of £400 per annum (£10,380), whilst the head teacher in the massage school was on a scale of £520-£600 (£13,599-£15,600). Six months later a Radiography Education and Welfare Sub Committee was appointed, reporting to the Nursing Committee. It was to include the Directors of the X-ray and Radiotherapy Departments, the Sister-in-Charge of each department, and the Lady Superintendent (the Matron) or her representative, the Chairman being one of the Directors. Selection of students would still be done by the Lady Superintendent who would also deal with disciplinary matters. It met for the first time on 22 April 1947, just a year before the National Health Service took over all responsibility for the hospital.

The war in Europe ended on 4 May 1945 and with Japan on 2 September 1945 and there was a determination to get life in the hospital and in the various medical educational establishments back to normal. On 16 May 1945 permission to un-brick the hospital windows was given. Two months later it was resolved that the physiotherapy school could return from Stoke Mandeville and that the Girl Guides who had been doing the washing up on the wards need no longer do so! There were no automatic dishwashers then. Presumably this latter course of action had been taken in part to deal with the crisis of lack of domestic staff. It was not until July 1946 that The Middlesex nursing staff and the Preliminary Training School were withdrawn from Stoke Mandeville Hospital. In September Mrs Clementine Churchill, wife of the war time Prime Minister, Winston Churchill, presented the prizes at the nurses' prize giving.

It was hoped that the bomb damage repairs would be completed by October 1947. York House, a nurses' home in Berners Street, had no heating because of a nationwide fuel crisis, and in September there was an emergency meeting because of an epidemic of infantile paralysis (now known as poliomyelitis). Twelve female students entered The Middlesex Hospital Medical School in 1947, the first time in the history of the school that women had been enrolled, sixty three years after the first medical school in the UK had admitted female students. This school was called the London School of Medicine for Women; it was established in 1874 and the students went to the Royal Free Hospital in Gray's Inn Road for their clinical training (it moved to Hampstead in the mid 1970s).

There was continuing concern over the hospital overdraft. In July it had been £117,134 (about three million pounds) with £90,000 being received from the Ministry of Health. Gifts of food were received from Australia and New Zealand as food rationing was still in place and extra supplies were always welcome.

In April 1948 arrangements were made for the final meeting of the Board of Governors. On 19 May the new Board under the NHS met, with Colonel John Jacob Astor elected as Chairman. The National Health Service now owned most hospitals in the country and became responsible for their financing and critically, debt. However, The Middlesex remained self-governing but under the aegis of the Department of Health. The Ministry exerted control over most aspects of hospital activities although private medicine still functioned, for in June it was resolved that every effort should be made to keep the Woolavington Wing (the private wing) free of ministerial control. Dr Graham Whiteside, a consultant in the x-ray department, reported that on the day that the NHS finally took over, a letter was received by the hospital that the shiny lavatory paper stamped with the NHS logo could now be used: control was being exerted down to the final undignified end.

With the war over, the students back at work in the main hospital, the National Health Service established, ordinary patients being diagnosed and treated, the x-ray and radiotherapy departments open for normal service, the education sub-committee set up, the lecture

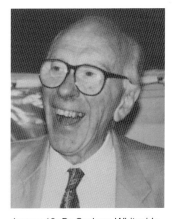

Image 18: Dr Graham Whiteside

programme and the process for appointment of lecturers agreed, it was time for the Schools to go forward, to develop and to begin to make their mark on the Radiographic world.

CHAPTER 2

Building a modern profession 1949 – 1979

In 1948, Sister Joan Parbery, a state registered nurse who had qualified as a radiographer, was both Superintendent of the Department and Principal of the School of Diagnostic Radiography. The qualification was still dual (Diagnosis and Therapy) and would remain so until 1951. Sister Mary Craig held similar positions in Radiotherapy and had done so since 1942. However, in 1948 Sister Parbery married and then took extended leave before giving in her notice. Marion Frank had qualified in 1941 at Glasgow Royal Infirmary and whilst employed as a Senior Radiographer at Derbyshire Royal Infirmary had taken an unpaid three-month post-diploma studentship at the Meyerstein Institute at The Middlesex Hospital, to increase her knowledge of radiotherapy practice before taking the Fellowship of the Society of Radiographers' examination (FSR). Her drive and determination were noted by both Professor Windeyer and Dr Graham Hodgson, and they were deeply impressed at her willingness to work unpaid in order to gain the experience she felt she needed. When the post of Superintendent and Principal in the Diagnostic department became available, Marion was working in Canada, and Professor Windeyer wrote to her suggesting she should apply for the post. Also at his suggestion, before returning to England she visited hospitals in New York, including the Mayo Clinic, specifically to investigate automatic processing installations. She returned to England for the interview, and was offered the post, which she accepted, the first person not already qualified as a nurse to be appointed to such a role at The Middlesex. Her salary was £521 (£11,900) per annum, with London weighting of £30 (£683), the latter amount being awarded because of the extra expense of living in the capital.

Although a structured syllabus for the radiography course had been devised by Sisters Parbery and Craig, course delivery was random, the lectures being given when the departments were not busy and the lecturers and space were available. The course as defined comprised lectures in Anatomy, Physics, Photography, Apparatus Construction and Radiographic Technique and Radiotherapy (see Appendix A). By the end of the two-year course the necessary lectures had usually been given but in modern terms it would seem haphazard. Students spent three-month periods alternating between the two departments (diagnosis and therapy) in order to gain the necessary practical experience. In 1951 the qualifications for radiotherapy and radiodiagnosis (x-ray) were separated, with a two year course required for each. Dual qualification was possible with a further twelve months' work (later to become eighteen months), students attending both first and second year lectures in the other discipline while doing clinical work in the appropriate department, gaining the same number of clinical examinations as the other students.

The arrival of Marion Frank in 1949, 'blew a fresh wind through the School' (Geraldine Stevenson), as she focused on her aim of developing it into one of the best education centres for radiographers in the country. The lecture programme was set up properly and rigorously adhered to, with defined hours of lectures in the week. There was an insistence on solid learning of the theoretical aspects which was closely linked with the practical experience. It was the beginning of the treatment of radiography students as students rather than apprentices who

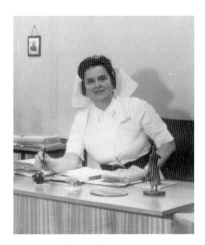

Image 19: Marion Frank

learnt on the job and whose first responsibility was to the needs of the department. Marion Frank and Mary Craig tried to ensure that the lecture programme met syllabus requirements, and that the demands of the clinical departments did not place the students' course at risk; at the same time great attention was paid to care for the patient, communication, technical expertise, and practical skills.

For radiotherapy students, clinical assignments were carried out throughout the department, including the treatment units, the isotope department (later to become nuclear medicine), treatment planning, the department office, observing preparation of radium applicators for theatre and local treatments, clinics, including departmental progress clinics which included ward rounds, outpatients, and those combined with the ear, nose and throat department. The placement period increased as students gained experience, certain areas being visited only in the final year. In addition students spent two weeks on the wards in order to understand ward routine and how they functioned. Each student was issued with a Record of Practical Training from the Society/College of Radiographers which required the student to complete 600 treatment set-ups, some of which would be assisted, and in addition they were required to spend time in the other areas of the department. They had to record the patients treated under each treatment modality: Superficial, Deep and Megavoltage X-ray, Gamma Ray Beam, Unsealed Sources, Physics (which

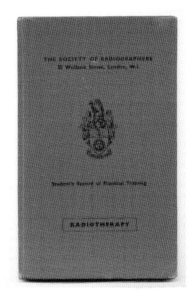

Image 20: Radiotherapy Logbook

encompassed treatment planning), Mould Room and Radium Department work, and Care of the Patient, both on the wards and in clinics. All this practical experience was verified at the time by a qualified radiographer and the book was signed by the Principal to indicate that the requisite tasks had been completed. This was then presented to the examiners at the viva voce examination. This practice ensured that the clinical radiographers were actively involved in the student's training. Students were advised not to put anything too complicated on the first page unless they were prepared for questions on the subject in the viva voce examination.

The diagnostic students were also allocated on a weekly basis to various investigation rooms in the x-ray department. In the early days these would include chest x-rays, intravenous pyelography (kidneys, ureters and bladder), spines and hips, extremities and casualty, barium enemas and meals, and mobile examinations (on the wards), as well as the darkroom and the office. As the students entered the second year they would add experience in dental examinations, tomography (sectional radiography), the skull room, including encephalography (an invasive x-ray examination of the ventricles of the brain starting with a lumbar puncture), and the 'specials' suite: arteriography (examination of the blood

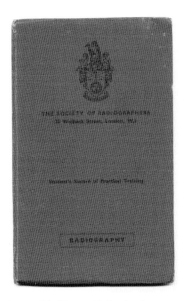

Image 21: Diagnostic Logbook

vessels), angiocardiography (examination of the heart), and the operating theatre, and after these developed, computerised tomography and radionuclide imaging. It was a rule, however, that students were not to go to post-mortems. When eighteen-year-old girls straight from school first started working on some of the examinations of a personal nature, such as barium enemas, hysterosalpingograms and male urethrograms, these could present something of a surprise or even shock. A Record of Practical Training similar to that for radiotherapy had to be completed. This defined by anatomical area the minimum number of patients a student had to have examined during their training.

The Schools introduced outside visits to manufacturers and to specialist hospitals to broaden and deepen the students' understanding of the treatment and imaging process. In the early days the radiotherapy students went to Mount Vernon Hospital in Northwood for experience in teletherapy and the use of the linear accelerator to extend their experience of different techniques. They also went on a number of day visits to other hospitals' departments, which included St Bartholomew's, to see patients receiving treatment in the cylindrical hyperbaric oxygen tank. In the early days of oxygen therapy the students visited St Thomas', where a converted deep sea diving bell was used for their oxygen tank, the patient being treated through the port-holes, which entailed wriggling up and down until they were in the correct spot! They went to St Luke's Hospital, Guildford, to see the Betatron, the Hammersmith Hospital to observe use of the Cyclotron for neutron therapy, and to the Royal Marsden, Fulham Road, to see the Van der Graph generator used for therapy treatment. Radiotherapy students went to some of the equipment manufacturers, including MEL (Mullard Electronics Ltd, which later became part of Philips) at Three Bridges, in Surrey, and TEM at Crawley (later part of Varian), where their treatment machines were being constructed. A favourite with the students was the visit to the atomic reactor at Harwell, where they were taken onto the platform above the reactor and were also shown equipment for remote handling of radioactive sources, decontamination equipment, 'space suit' protective clothing and monitoring equipment.

From the 1950s diagnostic students, in addition to their normal rotations, spent two weeks on the wards in order to understand how they functioned, and to spend a little more time with patients whom they would normally only see for a few minutes. They also went to the records department to aid understanding of the way record-keeping worked and the importance of accurate filing – in those days, of course, everything was paper-driven as there were no computers. There was a fortnight's course at Kodak Education Centre on Kingsway, which covered most of the photography syllabus, and which the students loved, as lunches and cakes for afternoon tea were provided and this eased personal budgets, and a day at the factory at Harrow, where the large site is now completely empty as photographic film is no longer needed. It was a similar situation for the revision courses at Ilford's Education Centre on Tavistock Square, before both the Part 1 and Part 2 qualification examinations. There were visits to the Dean factory in Croydon, to the Picker factory (later part of the General Electric Company) at North Wembley to see x-ray equipment and grids being made, and to be told that Picker liked employing Indian ladies for the making of grids, as they were

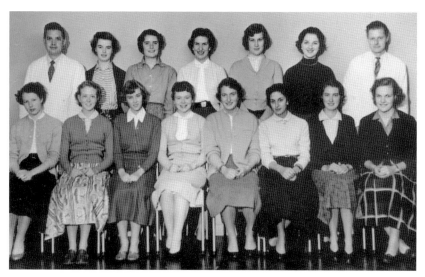

Image 22: Kodak Course 1956

much more painstaking and accurate than others; to Mullards to watch x-ray tubes being hand-made by the glass blowers; to the Science Museum to look at the history of the discovery of both electricity and x-rays. They also went to the dental department at The Middlesex, and to Queen Charlotte's Hospital at Hammersmith for experience in obstetric radiography.

In May 1962 Mr William Stripp, always known as Bill, the Superintendent Radiographer at the Royal National Orthopaedic Hospital, Great Portland Street, agreed to take Middlesex students for two weeks each in their senior year. Bill was an inspirational teacher, and it was the start of a very happy relationship, much enjoyed by the students and appreciated by the teaching staff. Bill Stripp was acknowledged world-wide as the expert in Orthopaedic Radiography. He was an artist in radiography and could image the most deeply concealed of bony conditions. He understood bony anatomy and its variations better than most, and he knew all the standard projections and could adapt them in an infinite variety of ways. He would sit with the most junior of students and give one-to-one tutorials until even they understood. When he died in 1988 a College of Radiographers' annual lecture was founded in his honour.

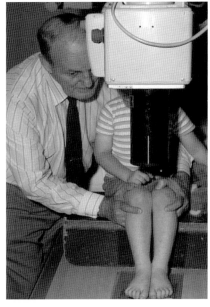

The course length for each discipline remained at two years until 1982, and dual qualification could still be obtained by studying for an extra eighteen months. There was a strong endeavour at this time to lift morale and increase pride in the Schools. Students were expected to pass both state and hospital examinations, although not everyone did. Those who did pass received hospital badges with their names engraved on the back, worn with pride throughout their professional life. The hallmark blue blazers with the Middlesex crest on the pocket were another equally-valued item of uniform.

Image 23: William (Bill) Stripp

Initially accommodation was not provided, and those unable to live at home had to find their own in residential clubs or hostels around London, as difficult to find then as it is now. At the beginning there was not even a canteen for lunch or coffee breaks. However, the Board of Governors under the Chairmanship of Lord Astor of Hever was well aware of the problems of accommodation for staff and were taking steps to try to obtain somewhere for non-nursing staff to live. Lord Astor had donated the money for the Nurses' home before the war but non-nurses could not live there. The Board's deliberations and negotiations finally culminated in the purchase of Marlborough Court, which cost £138,000 (£3.15 million). Marlborough Court was on the easterly end of a terrace in Lancaster Gate, its rooms overlooking Hyde Park on the south side and Lancaster Gate on the north, and it was first used in 1949.

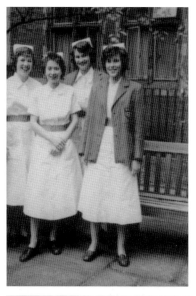

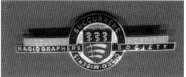

Image 24: The blue blazer & the hospital badge

There were initially thirty double rooms and ninety-six singles giving space for 156 residents. En suite facilities were not available. Fees charged to residents were £2 5s - £3 (£50-£68) per week for single occupancy for bed and breakfast and £1 15s - £2 5s (£40-£50) for shared occupancy, the latter option used by the majority of students. No unmarried men were allowed to live there. Despite representations to Matron from consultants in the hospital, members of the opposite sex were not allowed to be entertained in the rooms, although they were allowed in the lounge up to 11pm.

In July 1950 there was discussion as to whether a charge of 6d (60p) per week should be levied for 'wireless sets' used in their rooms by residents, presumably because of the cost of electricity, but it was thought to be too difficult to monitor.

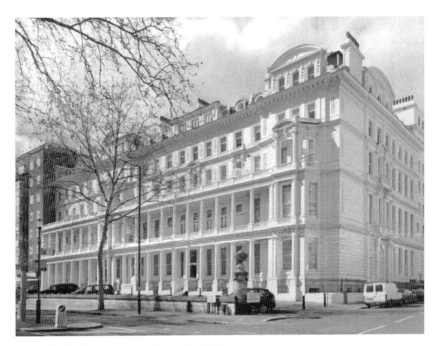

Image 25: Marlborough Court, Lancaster Gate

At the same time the installation of a bar was authorised and in May 1951 the purchase of a television set was agreed at a cost of £73 10s (£1700); in September a public telephone box was installed. None of these facilities had previously been available to residents, and there were certainly no telephones in the rooms. All these items would be regarded as necessities nowadays, but telephone lines at the time were 'rationed' and it was not uncommon to have to have a shared line in a private home. The cost of a television set was prohibitive for the ordinary person.

The role of warden was critical to the smooth running of the hostel, its financial viability, the catering, and by no means least, the happiness of the residents. Miss Barnes (no one seems to know her first name, and there is no written record that can be found) was appointed as resident secretary in February 1950 and remained there until it closed. Her annual salary was £500 (£11,400) plus board and lodging. The women who managed the reception were said to be a wonderful source of knowledge, information and advice, especially to young students living away from home for the first time.

John Twydle, who lived at Marlborough Court from 1972 to 1974, vividly remembers his time there:

'Marlborough Court was a key element of developing the 'Esprit de Corps' of the Schools (and the hospital). Many students lived there, especially in their first six months of training, alongside student teachers, Marion Frank, a long term resident from 1949 -1975, and a mixture of other professionals supplementary to medicine. There were doctors, physiotherapists, speech therapists, and many other ancillary staff. Located as it was on the edge of Hyde Park, it was a privilege to reside there. The rooms on the ground and first floors had tremendous height, maybe 12-14 ft (3.6-3.9m). Typical rooms on the ground floor were 24 ft (about 7m) long but these were subdivided and only 8-10 ft wide (2.5-3m). Two students would share such a room with a small basin for washing. Toilets and bathrooms were communal. On the south side the rooms facing the park were larger, especially on the first and second floors, and typically held three students or were single occupancy for qualified professionals.

'The communal bathrooms led to an incident when a radiologist managed to lock himself out of his room. Marion Frank was a neighbour and the radiologist knocked on Marion's door remembering that he had left his window open and that he and Marion shared a communal balcony. So that modesty could be preserved it was agreed through the door that Marion would open the door and then return to bed to hide under the covers. The radiologist entered, crossed the room, opened Marion's window and was about to exit when he trod on a mousetrap laid by Marion. The mousetrap snapped, the towel dropped and Marion emerged from the bedclothes to see what all the noise was about. Modesty was no longer preserved.

'When I started eleven of the fourteen students in my set were accommodated at Marlborough Court and my first room-mate was a Nigerian pharmacist whose eating habits I found challenging to live with; a quiet word to Marion and I was 'transferred' to share with the other male student in my set. From that moment on we became life-long friends. Life was never lonely, and one's ego was boosted significantly by taking nine ladies (my fellow students) to the pub round the corner. Often when one *or other of the set was down they could always look for support, advice or simply a cup of tea from one of the others in the group. It is a mark of the friendships built that thirty nine years later I am still in touch with about half of my set.*

'There was also a small kitchen on each floor where simple meals could be prepared. There was a communal dining room where most took breakfast and a few chose to have dinner. It was common for the toasting machine to get stuck, cremate some bread and set off the fire alarms. Apart from the sitting room in the entrance hall there was also a TV room and with such a wide variety of people and cultures there was rarely agreement on which channel to watch. The fact that you got to know colleagues outside work made for a stronger bond inside work. You would run into people around the hospital you knew and as such you were part of the wider team. Students and sometimes staff would often 'bounce back' to Marlborough Court when other living arrangements fell through or leases were unexpectedly terminated.

'There were a limited number of parking spaces secured by chain and padlock at the front of the property. There was a long waiting list for places but most people travelled by tube so places did occasionally become free. To have a room in such a delightful part of London with secure parking was a luxury few of us appreciated fully at the time.'

For many years Marlborough Court was used as the venue for The Society of Radiographers Annual Radiotherapy Weekend, a national meeting attracting radiotherapy radiographers from all over the United Kingdom. It was an ideal venue as it was in Central London and was within easy travelling distance of most main line stations.

Graham Buckley, the then Secretary-Superintendent (Chief Executive), said 'Marlborough Court was a successful venture and despite the restrictions became a much appreciated lodging for many hospital staff. For more than thirty years, under the administration of capable Wardens, it was a valued part of The Middlesex organisation. Following yet another review of the National Health Service, it was sold in 1980 - a matter of regret to many'.

The Fellowship (FSR) examination (to become the Higher Diploma (HDSR) in 1968) was instituted in November 1949, and Muriel Guest, a senior radiographer and deputy tutor was one of the first radiographers to pass in 1950. This started a tradition of clinical radiographers from The Middlesex passing their higher professional examinations, which continued until the advent of university education. Initially, department staff were expected to deliver lectures on clinical radiography as part of their role. The lecturers were reported as being excellent and were remembered as a very inspiring group of professionals, working hard with little or no remuneration for lecturing, and no time allowance for lesson preparation or for marking. Later,

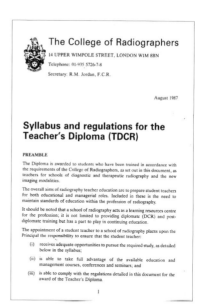

Image 26: Teacher's Diploma of the College of Radiographers

one or two were appointed as 'assistant tutors' giving them an allowance of £50 (£1,150) per year above their salary; it was expected that anyone appointed to this role would sit the Fellowship examination, and certainly the preparation of lectures was an excellent means of ordering one's thoughts and learning the basics.

The Teachers' Endorsement (TE) was introduced in 1956/1957, but it could only be taken if the lecturer already held the Fellowship. What the rules were initially is not known, but by 1963 the lecturer had to be able to lecture in five out of the six subjects required for qualification, and the examination consisted of a one hour lecture to a set of students unknown to the examiners, on a topic chosen by the candidate out of four subjects set by the examiners. Two examiners, one radiologist and one senior tutor radiographer, sat at the back of the classroom listening to the lecture and marked the teacher's performance. This was followed by a one hour tutorial, a question and answer session with the same students on any of the four topics. Having survived this ordeal candidates were then subjected to a forty-minute viva voce examination, where they could be asked any question on the subject of teaching and running a school of radiography. The last Teachers' Endorsement examination in this format was held in 1967, and was replaced the following year by the Teachers'

Diploma of the Society of Radiographers (TDSR). This qualification had much the same examination, but by then there was a requirement that the candidate spend a year as a student teacher in a recognised school, gain the City and Guild's Further Education Teacher's Certificate (FETC) and complete a logbook of their teaching experience. It became essential that candidates knew off by heart the content of all the many Training Centre (TC) documents. These were issued, from 1973 onwards, by the Society and subsequently the College of Radiographers and were the rules which 'had to be obeyed' by teachers and schools. The Fellowship was not an easy examination, with all subjects having to be passed simultaneously. By 1961 twenty radiographers from The Middlesex had passed it, and ten had gained the Teachers' Endorsement. In 1965 there were thirty-three entries from throughout the UK; there were eleven passes, five of them from The Middlesex School.

This was a period of consolidation for the Schools and for rapidly increasing work in both departments. There were now sixteen students admitted to the diagnostic school per year, with a two-year waiting list; radiotherapy had twelve places a year, four of which were for qualified nurses. The Middlesex Schools were reported as being among the largest in the country.

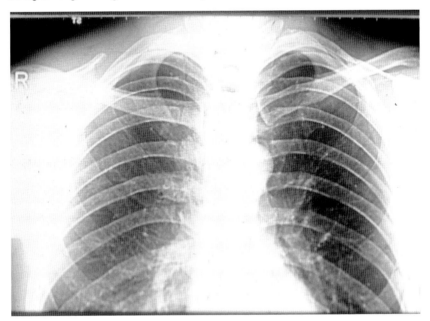

Image 27: Chest x-ray

From 1952 there was a steady increase in work to provide clinical experience for the students, only hampered by a shortage of x-ray film. There were ten x-ray rooms plus a room for angiocardiography, run by Geraldine Stuart (Stevenson), who had been one of the students in 1939. A mass miniature chest x-ray machine had been installed, meaning that every patient had a chest x-ray on admission, and by 1957, all hospital staff and medical students had a chest x-ray every six months; all pregnant women had one, as did all members of a family hoping to emigrate to Australia. The staff in the chest x-ray room were performing over a hundred examinations a day; as yet the concern over the risk of induction of cancer by the frequency with which people were exposed to low doses of radiation was not in evidence. In 1955, the year Sir Harold Graham Hodgson retired, the x-ray department had examined 71,000 patients, using 177,000 films. Sir Harold had been made a KCVO in 1950 for 'continued service to the Royal Family', having first examined King George V in 1929. Amazingly, the Schools still did not have a separate budget from the clinical departments; they were in competition with clinical needs, and had to apply for funds whenever equipment or books were needed. There was pressure on the Schools to take overseas post-qualification radiographers for the higher qualifications and for clinical experience, but any increase in numbers beyond those already existing could not take place until the issue of space was resolved.

In 1953, before male students were admitted, before the school had expanded into delivery of post-qualification courses to UK radiographers, and before large scale education was delivered to international qualified radiographers, a detailed report of the difficulties caused by the cramped conditions was given to the Hospital's House Committee. The following year Sister Mary Craig, Superintendent Tutor to the Radiotherapy Department and School, was elected Vice-President of the Society of Radiographers, and in 1957 to the Presidency, increasing her workload, and the need for space both for herself and for the many official visitors engendered by the office, not to mention the rising tide of paperwork and file space associated with the post.

In 1963 there were thirty two diagnostic and twenty four radiotherapy students. The School accommodation comprised a classroom for twenty five, a small study room, a sitting room for six which doubled as a study room, and a locker room shared with the physiotherapy students and records staff. Apart from the classroom, which was underneath the front car park and was therefore very dark with little natural light, the other facilities were on the basement corridor of the x-ray department, opposite three heavily-used clinical rooms which had no waiting accommodation or dressing rooms. The corridor was a very busy through route, with lots of noisy trolleys, and lined with patients in wheel-chairs, some of them very ill, awaiting x-ray. There was no accommodation for teachers, and no demonstration room or facilities for practical instruction. The Principal of the Diagnostic Radiography School was still also the Superintendent and had a small office, shared with her deputy. It contained all the records and correspondence, and doubled as their changing room and uniform store. The room had also to be used for interviewing, discussion and counselling. A further problem was that the Principal of the Radiotherapy School was based at the other side of the hospital in similar accommodation in the West Wing, a good five minute walk away. This did not aid a co-ordinated approach for the two Schools.

The minimum requirements for the two schools were listed as follows in the report presented to the Hospital's planning committee in November 1953:

i.   An office for each Superintendent/Tutor
ii.   An office for the other tutors
iii. Two classrooms, one for sixty students and one for fifteen
iv.   Library/study/film viewing room for thirty with viewing boxes
v.   Demonstration and practical classroom
vi.   Sitting room
vii. Cloakroom with sixty or seventy lockers
viii. Cupboards for books
ix.   Lavatories and washroom

Amazingly, by 1957 only a small amount of further space for the School had been acquired. There were now two classrooms, and forty desks and sixty chairs had been bought. It was still insufficient, with four sets of students in both diagnosis and radiotherapy for the two-year training, with a further two sets for about three months when there was an overlap of courses. There was a room which had multiple uses as a reference library, film viewing room, a small museum of apparatus, and for study. It was also occasionally used for tutorials. Quiet study for students was impossible and there was nowhere for staff to prepare lectures.

The need for office space for school staff had not been addressed. Four years later, in 1961, it was reported that a classroom and a small tutor's room had been taken over by the x-ray department to accommodate an Image Intensifier room, giving even less space to the school: educational needs were overwhelmed by clinical requirements. The toilets were shared by forty-three staff, forty students, eleven office staff, three darkroom technicians and ten physiotherapists. The student changing area was again shared and overcrowded in the basement of outpatients, a ten minute walk away via the creepy underground tunnels. An application was again made for additional accommodation, and was again ignored by the planning committee. In 1963 Marion Frank stressed again the urgency of a move to give more space for the current situation, as well as to allow the Schools to expand and deliver courses to international radiographers.

The interest in international radiography had started very early in the Department's life. Sir Harold Graham Hodgson had quickly built up and maintained the department's reputation for teaching radiologists and it became one of the foremost centres for postgraduate radiological instruction in the country. Where overseas radiologists trained in their speciality, they often recommended the department to their radiographers when they, in their turn, sought higher qualifications. At the end of 1952 Marion Frank and Mary Craig applied for study leave to attend the International Congress of Radiology (ICR) in Copenhagen and to visit departments in Stockholm and Germany. It was an undoubted advantage to The Middlesex team that Marion Frank spoke fluent German and French. There would be a big exhibition of equipment to look at with a view to purchases for the x-ray and radiotherapy departments, but it was also an excellent opportunity for them to meet experts from overseas, to network and to discuss ideas. Additionally, Professor Windeyer wanted Mary Craig to visit the United States to investigate how forward-thinking departments were equipping and planning for the future. Clinical radiographers were already gaining experience abroad. Experienced radiographers went from The Middlesex to the Republic of South Africa, to Canada and to Singapore in 1955, and in 1959 a diagnostic radiographer, Wendy Lowe, went to Massachusetts General Hospital in Boston as Tutor in Charge. Marion Frank again visited the ICR in Munich in 1959 and it was at this meeting that the idea of setting up an International Society of Radiographers was first mooted. It was to become the International Society of Radiographers and Radiological Technicians (ISRRT), the term Technicians later being changed to Technologists, and she and Kathleen Clark, who had originally encouraged Marion Frank to become a radiographer, became founder members.

Visitors came to the school from the United States, Nigeria, Canada and New Zealand. In December 1961 it was reported to the Education Committee that the World Health Organisation (WHO) had approached Professor Windeyer to ask him if The Middlesex could offer overseas radiographers post-diploma courses leading to the Fellowship, organise and provide experience in modern radiography, and help them develop towards future leadership roles. This was agreed, despite the lack of space. They were to be offered attendance at lectures, use of library and study facilities, and observation of special techniques, and arrangements would be made for them to visit specialist hospitals. They were to be charged at the rate of ten guineas (£10 10s: worth £160 in 2005) per quarter. In 1965 there were six overseas students studying for the Fellowship, two of them being pupil teachers, from Ethiopia, Nigeria, Jamaica, Hong Kong and Barbados and World Health had sponsored a radiographer from Singapore. These still had to be fitted into the inadequate space previously described and there was an undoubted and increasing demand for post-qualification education and experience. Marion Frank attended the West African radiological meeting in Lagos and represented the United Kingdom at the ISRRT meetings in place of Kathleen Clark, who was ill. A year later, Marion was elected to the Council of the ISRRT and became Junior Vice-President of the Society of Radiographers.

In 1966 Professor Sir Brian Windeyer was scheduled to discuss the increased facilities needed for the postgraduate courses with the Ministry of Overseas Development, the Council of Europe, the World Health Organisation and the British Council. Perhaps these high-powered discussions finally drove The Middlesex Hospital's planning committee to make a decision to allow the enlargement of the Schools. At last, in 1966 and at relatively short notice, Marion Frank and Mary Craig were informed by the planning officer that most of Doran House in Foley Street would be allocated to the school and that they should produce plans (no budget and no expert advice) as to how they would use it. Doran House was an old warehouse and not easy to plan. There were enormous square load-bearing columns, measuring at least thirty by thirty centimetres, which appeared destined to be right in the middle of classrooms. Staff, unsurprisingly, unskilled in such planning, spent fruitless effort and time trying to see how to make a modern

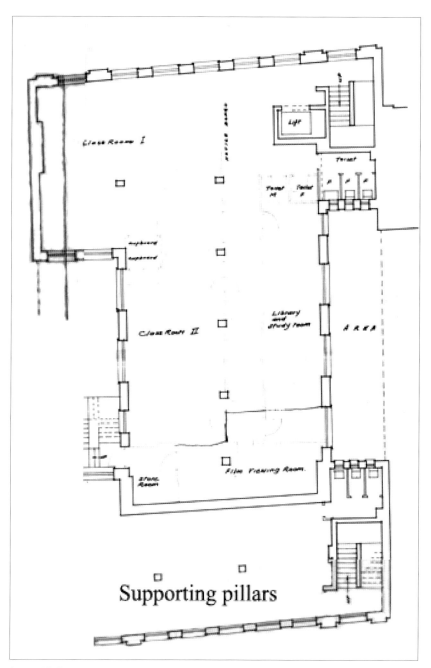

Image 28: Doran House - plan of the second floor

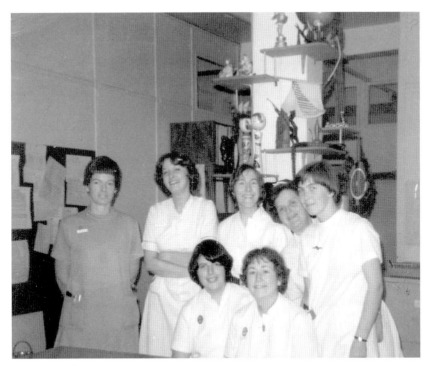

Image 29: Reception area column: Back row Anne Wells, Christine Gill, Adrienne Finch, Marion Frank, Mary Embleton; Front row: Julia Lovell, Margaret McClellan

education centre out of a warehouse. Finally Alan Penney, the architect husband of a past Deputy Principal of the Diagnostic School, June Penney (Legg), produced an excellent outline which was workable.

The first and second floors of Doran House backed on to the catering and domestic services departments, and most of the ground floor and the entire basement were engineering and carpentry departments, which was very useful when students lost their locker keys and padlocks had to be sawn off! Additionally most of the conversion work was done at cost by the engineering department. The rest of the building, totalling four floors, was allocated to the Radiography Schools. The entrance lobby and cloakroom for outdoor clothes was on the ground floor. The first floor had a large open-plan reception and administration area, staff offices, the two Principals' offices, a library for post-diploma and postgraduate students, and a staff changing room. The load bearing column

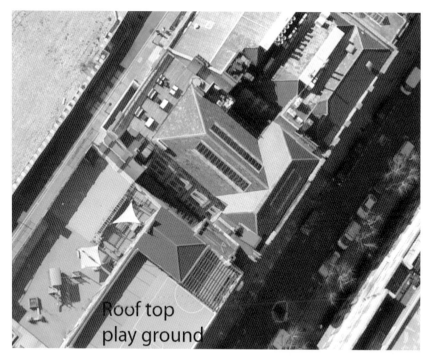

Image30: All Souls' Primary School's rooftop playground and the adjacent rooftop terrace of the Schools of Radiography

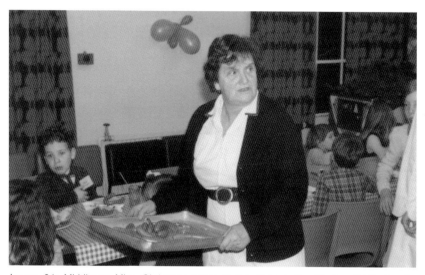

Image 31: Middlesex Mice Christmas party in the School. Frankfurter distribution by Marion Frank.

immediately in front of the reception desk became a feature, its shelves loaded with many unusual pieces of craft work donated by post diploma students and visitors from all over the world.

There were two big classrooms on the second floor, connected by storage cupboards with sliding doors on either side, from which Marion Frank used secretly to oversee new teachers, emerging like a genie at the lecture end with appropriate comments. There was also an L-shaped library, which overlooked All Souls' primary school next door and was not the best place to try and study when the children were on their rooftop playground. The third floor had locker rooms for female staff and students, practical classrooms for diagnostic and radiotherapy students, a photographic dark room and a store.

The main feature of the fourth floor was the large common room, with a separate kitchen and a roof terrace, much used in the summer. This area was the venue of the Schools' famed social events, including the annual Christmas Lunch and the Mouse Parties. The Middlesex Mice were founded well before World War II and to be a member you had to be a child of a member of staff. It was primarily a fund-raising group for the paediatric ward. There was also a radiologists' study room and male locker rooms. For staff used to being in incredibly cramped conditions the space provided was unbelievable.

The Schools moved into their new accommodation in Foley Street early in 1967 and a big party was held that summer to celebrate; the building was formally opened on 5 December 1967 by Lord Cobbold, the Chairman of the Board of Governors at The Middlesex, in the presence of the Secretary of the Society of Radiographers, representatives of the Ministry of Health, the Ministry of Overseas Development and the Royal College of Radiologists.

Up to this point the Diagnostic and Therapy Schools' administration had functioned separately with limited space available for School staff in the individual departments. Not only did the new accommodation bring both Schools under one roof, but the administration of the Schools was also adjacent on the first floor. Ann Paris and Christine Soutter, diagnostic and radiotherapy teachers respectively, shared an office directly behind Marion Frank's office, although subsequently they had separate space. Apart from better integration of the two Schools' staff, the diagnostic and radiotherapy students were able to understand each others' points of view better as they shared lecture rooms, study facilities, common rooms and changing rooms. At last the Schools were able take male students, never previously allowed because of the lack of a cloakroom and toilets. It enabled the development of a more formal programme in preparation for FSR/HDSR, and the possibility of training teachers on secondment from other centres. It was also possible to expand the post-diploma work and, critically, the number of international students, for which there was a particular demand from individual governments, and also from the World Health Organisation (WHO). In the days of apartheid, it was good to see a white South African and a black Ugandan walking down Oxford Street, sharing an umbrella.

With the closer co-operation between the Schools it was possible to organise postgraduate courses for the Fellowship Examination for both disciplines; the participants were not only the Schools' postgraduate students but radiographers from other hospitals who wanted to prepare for the examination. It was the first time a Fellowship course had been run which included subjects for radiotherapy radiographers.

In March 1969 there was a Teachers' Seminar in Copenhagen organised by the International Society of Radiographers and Radiological Technicians, and Marion Frank was very keen that as many of the overseas postgraduate students as possible would give papers at this meeting. For some this was not easy and they needed a lot of assistance, which meant several long evenings spent providing help and encouragement. This was probably one of the first occasions when the new kitchen on the fourth floor was put through its paces; the menus were varied, particularly when one of the overseas students was the cook. On occasions there was a trade-off, the student cooked whilst the member of staff got their paper ready for presentation! Other times it was just a willing soul, Mary Medhurst (Pluister) from Canada would regularly be heard muttering about this strange British custom of warming the plates! On one occasion there was a discussion regarding the menu; Marion had suggested a stuffed chicken, but Christine Soutter commented she did not like anything which had been inside a bird. Marion's quick reply was "you eat eggs; just think where they've been!"

The seminar was a great success: all the papers were delivered very professionally and gave a great personal boost, particularly to those speaking in public for the

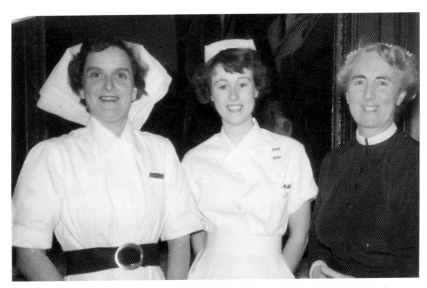

Image 32: A prize winning student with Marion Frank and Marjorie Marriott (Matron)

first time and in the majority of cases not in their mother tongue. The long evenings and the varied meals had not been in vain.

Up to 1965 the person responsible for the Schools had been the Matron, Marjorie Marriott, and the administration and admission of students had been done by the Matron's office. Student admission offers had been signed by the Matron and the Principals had presented her with a weekly report. In 1965, close to retirement, Miss Marriott asked to be relieved of this responsibility. It was suggested that the director of each department be Head of School, and that the Radiographic Committee be represented on the Nursing Committee by the director of the department or his deputy, with the Principals having the same status as Assistant Matrons. The Radiography Schools were now the responsibility of the medically qualified radiologists and radiotherapists, in place of the nurse administration, but not radiography tutors, so the two Principals were still not formally in charge.

In 1968 discussions were started with St Mary's Hospital, Paddington, on the possibility of some form of linkage which would allow The Middlesex diagnostic students access to the clinical department at St Mary's, as it was difficult to provide sufficient clinical experience at The Middlesex for the large number of students. There was supposed to be some practical teaching carried out by the radiographers responsible, and there had to be someone formally designated as a supervisor (there was no tradition of student radiographers at St Mary's) and in some cases radiographers had chosen to work there because there were no students. Initially there was a hope, never to be realised, that there could be a joint school, allowing an increase of numbers with a tutor appointed to St Mary's. The talks broke down through financial problems, but secondment of two senior students for two months each was negotiated, the agreement to be reviewed in two years. The students really enjoyed their time there, but no formal instruction was available, and as the

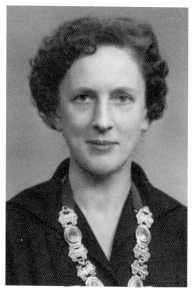

Image 33: Mary Craig

senior radiographer responsible had left, there was no-one in charge of them. In 1975 the radiotherapy students were seconded to St John's Hospital for Diseases of the Skin, in Soho, for experience in the treatment of skin tumours.

In 1972, at last, there was discussion on the separation of the budgets of the Schools and the departments, so that the Schools actually were able to spend money on books and teaching aids instead of having to be in competition with clinical needs which tended to win out. In July 1974 the budget was £30,516 (about £313,000 in today's figures).

i.	Diagnostic student bursaries	£21,928
ii.	Books	£150
iii.	Teaching aids	£330
iv.	Therapy bursaries	£7,828
v.	Books	£150
vi.	Teaching aids	£130

However, the problem of not knowing how much would be required for student bursaries was ongoing. The bursaries were awarded according to parental

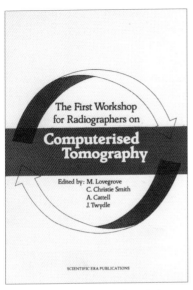

The First Workshop for Radiographers on

Computerised Tomography

Edited by: M. Lovegrove
C. Christie Smith
A. Cattell
J. Twydle

SCIENTIFIC ERA PUBLICATIONS

Image 34: Proceedings of workshop on computerised tomography

means, which could not be predicted, and in 1975 the diagnostic bursary budget was overspent by one third. Nor was it known how many students would be recruited before the budget was set, although the Radiotherapy School was now having problems getting enough students.

In 1974, The Society of Radiographers brought in regulations that stated that a full-time Principal must be appointed, and that anyone intending to take the Teachers' examination must be appointed full-time and for a minimum period of one year to a School of Radiography. Marion Frank and Mary Craig were both 50% Principals and 50% Superintendents.

So, in September 1975 Marion Frank became the full-time Principal and gave up her role in the department, and Jean Harvey became Superintendent of the X-ray department. Mary Craig retired in 1974 and a new Principal of the School of Radiotherapy, Anne Wells, was appointed as well a new Superintendent, Margaret Wells (they were not related).

Wherever there was a demand for increased knowledge for both clinical and education staff in a particular sphere or there was a need for some specialist knowledge by the many international students, a course would be run whether for a day, a weekend, or even longer. Hence there was a two-week course on the use of the overhead projector (up to that time the only visual aid was the blackboard). This course recruited twenty-one radiographers from thirteen countries. There was a course on teaching radiation physics by practical experiment and in 1980 a seven day workshop on Computer Tomography took place. A write-up of the proceedings was published and was so popular that £300 (£3,000) in royalties came into the Schools. In 1981 a course was run on quality assurance and control (QA). For this the clinical department was used and there was heavy involvement of the clinical staff. Later on, in 1985, there was a highly successful course on 'Writing for the Profession'.

Change was taking place in the Radiotherapy Department with the retirement of Sir Brian Windeyer at the end of 1969. He had been appointed to be in charge of the department on 1 January, 1936, he had been Medical Commandant of the Hospital during the war, was appointed a Professor of the University of London in 1942, and was Dean of the Medical School from 1954 to 1967. He had been an enormous and very influential supporter of the Schools. Margaret Snelling took over as Director of the Radiotherapy Department and School, Dr Margaret Spittle was appointed Consultant Radiotherapist and Norman Bleehen became Professor, only to move to Cambridge in 1975, when he

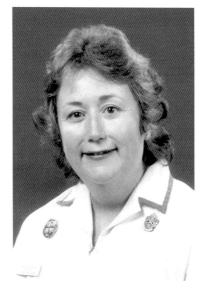

Image 35: Margaret McClellan

was replaced by Professor Roger Berry. Professor Berry had a particular interest in Radiobiology and in educating radiographers, and was soon involved in the School, giving lectures to the students on the biological effects of radiation; he would inform them that, if there were a nuclear incident, they would be experts. When Margaret Snelling retired he became Director of the Radiotherapy School.

In 1979, the College of Radiographers discovered that The Middlesex School had no College representative on its committee, nor had it ever been inspected. This oversight had possibly been caused by Marion Frank's position and the high reputation of the School. However, it was known that Marion was retiring the following year and action had to be taken. Nowadays the amount of effort and stress produced by inspections is well known, but then it was new to the staff. An enormous amount of paperwork was generated, and a large amount of cleaning, clearing out and tidying up done. The School passed with flying colours, and a College representative was appointed. Anne Wells retired and Mary Embleton, a former student and student teacher at The Middlesex, became Radiotherapy Principal. Marion Frank retired and Margaret McClellan, who had trained as a radiography teacher at The Middlesex, was appointed in her place. The next era had begun.

CHAPTER 3

Technical Innovation 1895 – 1991

At the same time as the Schools were developing at The Middlesex Hospital, the practice of radiography and radiotherapy was changing. Technical innovation was gathering pace, enlarging and extending the range and types of examinations and treatments, and in turn influencing the education of student radiographers, expanding the content of the syllabus leading to the implementation of three year training and increasing the demand for specialist post-diploma courses leading to formal qualifications. In some cases these technical innovations were the principal cause of diversity within the profession, with evolution into the worlds of Medical Ultrasound and Nuclear Medicine.

Radiotherapy

When it opened in 1938, the Meyerstein Institute of Radiotherapy was a state-of-the-art department. The equipment at the time consisted of five 200 kVp x-ray machines (known as Orthovoltage or Deep X-ray, DXR) which were used to treat the majority of patients. There were also two 100 kVp units, Superficial X-ray, SXR, and a unit for Teletherapy (where a radioactive source is at a distance from the patient), in this case at 8cm distance, and carried out with 5 grammes of radium. There were also facilities for treating patients with surface radium.

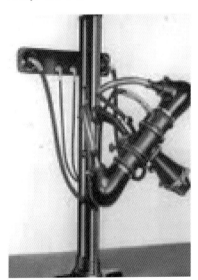

It was difficult, even when numerous fields from different directions were used, to deliver adequate absorbed doses to a deep seated tumour without at the same time delivering a high dose on the surface of each field, causing severe damage to the skin of the patient. With the 200 kVp machines the dose dropped to half that on the surface by about 6cms depth in the patient. What was needed

Image 36: Marconi Deep X-ray unit

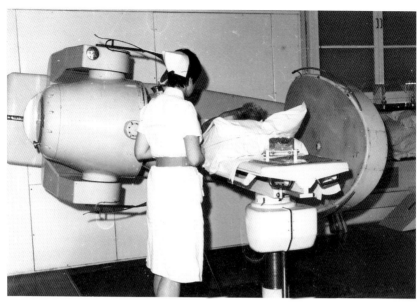

Image 37: Telecobalt unit

was a means of producing more penetrating beams without having to generate very high voltages.

There were two major breakthroughs in physics which led to the development of radiotherapy machines producing more penetrating beams of radiation. The first was the development of particle accelerators: the Betatron, developed by Donald W. Kerst in 1940, and the Van der Graff accelerator and the linear accelerator at around the same time. These provided a means of increasing the energy of electrons used to produce the x-rays, which meant the resultant x-ray beam was of higher energy and more penetrating and therefore more suitable for treating deep-seated tumours; it had the added advantage that the maximum dose was below the skin surface so patients did not get such severe skin reactions. These treatment machines were all big and cumbersome and needed a large area to accommodate them. Although they were being installed at other centres from the early 1950s, it was not until 1969, when further developments to the technology applied to Linear Accelerators had made them less bulky, that one was installed in the Meyerstein Institute. In the meantime the students were taught the theory, construction and use of them and visited other departments, including Mount Vernon Hospital, to gain practical experience.

The other development was that, as artificial isotopes of elements produced in nuclear reactors were becoming available, their potential for use in radiotherapy was being discovered. During 1951-1952 the idea of using caesium-137 for teletherapy was put forward by scientists at Oak Ridge in the United States, and at Harwell by those in the United Kingdom, and the UK Atomic Energy Authority developed a suitable caesium source. About this time Harold E. Johns in Canada invented cobalt-60 teletherapy. This development provided a tremendous boost in the quest for higher photon (X and gamma ray) energies and placed the cobalt unit at the forefront of radiotherapy for a number of years.

Each of these new treatment modalities produced beams that were more penetrating than conventional x-ray beams. The beam from caesium-137 was the least penetrating, but had the advantage that the radioactivity decayed slowly: it had a half life of 30 years compared with cobalt-60, whose half life was 5.25 years, and monthly adjustments needed to be made to treatment times, and the source needed replacing about every three years. A major problem was the comparatively large size of the source, meaning quite a high dose round the edge of the treatment beam giving irradiation to an unwanted area for the sake of the correct dose to the defined area. Margaret Wells, a student from 1948 to 1950, who worked in the Meyerstein Institute and later became Superintendent, recalled a problem with an early caesium unit in the Department. An error was made with the equipment whilst setting it up for a patient's treatment, which fortunately did not affect the patient, but revealed a design fault, and the machine had to be redesigned to make it foolproof. During the 1960s there were two caesium and two cobalt teletherapy units, but by the early 1970s the caesium units were being used very little and were phased out. The cobalt units were used predominantly for the treatment of patients with head and neck and breast tumours.

Technological advances in the design of Linear Accelerators (Linacs), which were used for treating deeper tumours in the pelvis and thorax, made them more compact and more efficient, and they were able to rotate round the patient. This allowed treatment from several directions, whilst focusing on the same point within the tumour, with the patient remaining in the same position, thus allowing structures closer to the skin surface of the patient to receive a lower dosage. This led to the first linear accelerator being installed at The Middlesex in 1969; it used 8 MeV (Mega electron volts) x-rays to treat patients.

The production of radioactive isotopes in the nuclear reactor also led to more suitable alternatives gradually replacing radium-226 (a naturally occurring radioactive isotope), for intracavity, interstitial (implanted directly into the tumour) and surface application. These isotopes meant less radiation risk should a source become lost or damaged, than from radium, with its half-life of 1620 years, and radioactive daughter products including the gas radon-222. Physicist Tom Bryant used to tell students about having to track rubbish collected from the hospital after discovering a patient had removed an interstitial radium needle and put it in the rubbish bag by his bed, and the 'lady from Soho' who discharged herself while being treated with intracavity gynaecological radium sources, and presumably returned to her profession, the applicators still in situ! Coupled with the introduction of new isotopes was the development of afterloading systems for Brachytherapy (where the radiation source is applied in or near the tumour) by remote means. Specifically-designed catheters could be inserted into the patient, their position radiographically checked and dosage calculation made prior to radioactive source(s) being loaded into the catheter and treatment given. This could also be used for surface application.

The Cathetron, which was introduced into the Meyerstein Institute at the beginning of the 1970s, used a remote control mechanism to drive the cobalt-60 sources from a shielded safe, and reduced the risk of unnecessary radiation exposure to the operator. This used a high dose rate, which meant treatment times were a few minutes compared with days when radium was used. As the Meyerstein Institute was one of the few departments to have a Cathetron, students from other schools visited to see it in operation.

In the early 1970s the use of the Linear Accelerator at The Middlesex extended to the use of electrons ranging from 3 -10 MeV. The machine could be switched from the x-ray treatment mode to the electron mode by removing the target the electrons hit to produce x-rays and placing a scattering foil to distribute the electrons across the desired area for treatment. Electrons, being particles, do not travel far in tissue and are used to treat tumours on or close to the skin with no dose to underlying structures. This removes the radiation risk to the operator that occurred with the surface application of sources, such as radium. The curriculum expanded to encompass these new technologies, how they worked, their relative uses, advantages and disadvantages and associated radiation protection.

The development of computers also made a large impact on radiotherapy. The first radiotherapy planning computer facility was installed at The Middlesex in 1970 but limited time 'on line' meant that much of the treatment planning was still done by hand. Planning computers soon became smaller and more sophisticated and computer planning became the norm. Although students started to learn computer planning, they still had to learn to plan by hand to understand the principles.

The development of Radiotherapy Treatment Simulators, constructed like a treatment machine but with a diagnostic x-ray tube and image intensification, allowed the treatment area to be located and radiographs taken with the patient positioned as they would be on the therapy machine. Prior to this, films had been taken with a mobile x-ray unit for location of the treatment volume, and

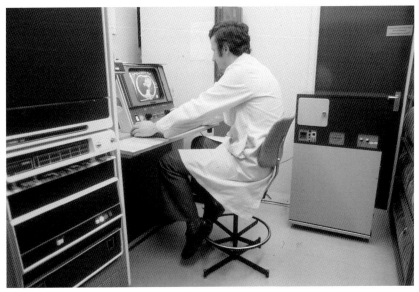

Image38: Radiologist review console CT 5005

on occasions in the x-ray department with a therapy radiographer present to ensure the patient was in the treatment position, which was invariably at odds with normal patient positioning. Development of Computerised Tomography (CT) and the location of a unit in the Meyerstein Institute in the late 1970s allowed cross sectional images to be produced with the patient in the treatment position, thus improving accurate localisation of the tumour. Planning computers were developed, which enabled the treatment dosimetry to be planned directly onto the CT image and show more accurately the dosage to the treatment volume and nearby sensitive organs.

Rapid advances were also being made in the development and use of cytotoxic (harmful to cells) drugs and chemotherapy using single agents or a combination of drugs being used alone or in association with radiotherapy and surgery. Students needed to have an overall knowledge of the management of cancer patients and a new subject entered the curriculum "Principles of Radiotherapy and Oncology" (see Appendix A).

Radionuclide imaging (RI)

In 1946 Professor John Eric Roberts had succeeded Professor Sidney Russ as Professor of Medical Physics, and at once saw that the long tradition of specialisation in radiation physics could be extended by exploiting for medical use the artificial radioactive isotopes of elements, which were at that time beginning to be available as a by-product of fission in nuclear reactors. A radioisotope laboratory was set up. By 1948 a limited diagnostic service using a small range of radioactive materials was available to The Middlesex Hospital. The service grew rapidly and soon the whole of the top floor of the Barnato-Joel Laboratories was being used for nuclear medicine diagnosis and research. It also became necessary for someone medically qualified to take a supervisory role and a registrar and nursing sister were seconded from the radiotherapy department.

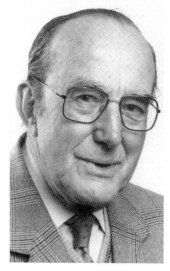

Image 39: Professor JE Roberts

85

By the late 1950s a significant proportion of the commitments of the physics department was devoted to the Isotope Diagnostic Service, and medical physics was also extending its frontiers. It was becoming involved with radiation safety, and quality control of equipment in x-ray, radiotherapy and anywhere electronic devices were used, and deserved the full attention of a professor with a complete staff of physicists. Thus the idea evolved for the creation of a new department, the sole work of which would be the provision of an isotope service in the broadest sense, which would also be an academic department of the Medical

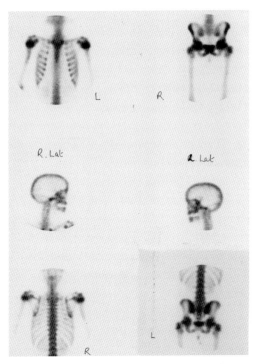

Image 40: A 1986 nuclear medicine scan using physiology to detect disease

School. Professor Brian Windeyer, as Dean of the Medical School, enthusiastically supported the proposal put forward by Professor Roberts, and the Institute of Nuclear Medicine was established in June 1961, as a new separate department. The Nuffield Foundation showed a particular interest in the project and provided a substantial grant for the Institute to be installed in a building specifically designed for the purpose. This was opened on 24 February 1969 by the Rt Hon. Lord Todd, FRS, though it had been occupied and had been providing a nuclear medicine service for a while.

The Institute of Nuclear Medicine had also been closely involved with the training of radiographers, and from the beginning, radiotherapy radiographers rotated in pairs for two periods of two weeks for the part of their training which related to the use of unsealed sources. Mary Embleton (Donaldson), who was a student from 1969 to 1971, remembers:

Sister Lillian Irene Pope was Superintendent of the Nuclear Medicine Department, and radiotherapy students spent the same amount of time there as on each of the placements within the Radiotherapy Department. Some of my fellow students found her intimidating. However, during one of my placements in Nuclear Medicine the department was exceptionally busy and one day I missed my lunch break. At the end of the week Sister Pope gave me a thank-you card signed by the staff, and a small gift. She was also the only person I remember discussing my report form with me as she filled it in, asking me how well I thought I had done and usually agreeing with my self-assessment.

The advent of computers, the development of the gamma camera, and the availability of a greater number of suitable isotopes for imaging meant that the scope of nuclear medicine had vastly increased, and in the early 1970s the Society of Radiographers started considering founding a qualification in Nuclear Medicine. Marilyn Swann (Walton) recalls:

Valerie Sharpe (Crown) had been running sessions for radiographers at the Royal Marsden School of Radiotherapy in Surrey, but once the Society said they wanted to have a Diploma, Marion Frank wanted The Middlesex to be the first school with a teacher qualified in Nuclear Medicine so that the school could run the first official course.

Marilyn Swann had just finished her diagnostic teacher training and did not need any persuading when Marion Frank suggested she should try for the Diploma in Nuclear Medicine. 'It was always easier to say Yes'. So she had to go and work in Nuclear Medicine, with 'Sister Pope in charge, very old fashioned, but a good sense of humour, a good old stick'. The theory was delivered on a day-release basis and there were a few evening sessions, organised mostly via Valerie Sharpe (Crown) and Dr Ralph McCready at the Royal Marsden. Marilyn sat and passed the first Diploma of Nuclear Medicine examination of the College of Radiographers. Marion Frank wanted a course set up for the following year, and Val Crown and Dr McCready agreed that the course should be conducted at The Middlesex, in liaison with the Royal Marsden Hospital, because of the premises and position: students came from all over London and the south-east of England. In 1976 the School of Nuclear Medicine was founded, with

Marilyn Swann as Principal, Professor Edward Williams as Director, and a part-time secretary, the course now being run solely by The Middlesex Hospital on a day release basis.

During the second half of 1970s the Institute of Nuclear Medicine acquired a new large field of view Anger Gamma Camera and associated computer system, a second small field of view camera and a dedicated SPET (Single Photon Emission Tomography) unit for tomography of the whole brain, and a dedicated SPET unit for tomographic studies of the whole body. SPET was the nuclear medicine equivalent of CT (computerised tomography) in radiography resulting in the production of cross sectional functional images of organs. New radiopharmaceuticals, radioisotopes in a chemical form or joined to a carrier, which can be used to assess the function of an organ or a physiological process, were also being developed, which increased the range of studies being performed.

Many hospitals without nuclear medicine departments started installing gamma cameras and facilities for preparing and administering radioactive isotopes for diagnostic investigations in x-ray departments. In 1981 the Nuclear Medicine qualification became the Diploma of Radionuclide Imaging, when the College of Radiographers decided to drop the therapy content and concentrate on the imaging aspects in the syllabus.

Medical Ultrasound (MUS)

In the early 1960s medical ultrasound was introduced to the imaging world. It was significant then because Alice Stewart's epidemiological research clearly indicated that x-raying a pregnant woman significantly increased the risk of the foetus subsequently developing leukaemia, and because ultrasound waves are non ionising and therefore do not have that risk, initially the modality was used primarily for imaging the foetus. Ultrasonography is the imaging of deep structures of the body by recording the echoes of pulsed ultrasound (U/S) waves directed into the patient's body which are then reflected by tissue planes where there is a change in density. These echoes are then converted into electrical impulses and displayed on a video display unit (VDU) presenting a 2D or 3D "picture". The ultrasound waves are produced by electrically stimulating a crystal called a transducer. It is excellent for differentiating between soft tissues which x-rays cannot and is good for examining the foetus, abdominal organs, heart and blood

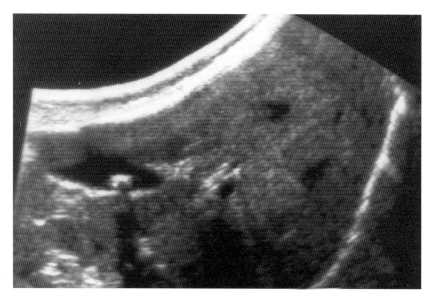

Image 41: An early ultrasound scan

vessels. However it cannot penetrate bone and is totally reflected by air so nothing can be imaged beyond bone or an air filled cavity. Doppler ultrasound scanning is a means to assess how substances, usually blood, flow. These results are displayed either graphically or as a colour image. The advent of the microchip in the late 1970s and subsequent increases in processing power have allowed the development of faster and more powerful systems and new ways of interpreting and displaying data.

In 1955 Professor Ian Donald was appointed Regius Chair of Midwifery at Glasgow University and led the pioneering work for developing ultrasound for medical use in the UK. His article 'Investigation of Abdominal Masses by Pulsed Ultrasound', published June 7, 1958 in the medical journal *The Lancet*, was one of the defining publications in the field. He had first explored the use of ultrasound after seeing it used in the Glasgow shipyards to look for flaws in metallurgy. Adrienne Finch has a clear memory of his giving a formal discourse at the Royal Institution (RI) in London on the subject. There has always been a tradition of practical demonstration at the RI and in his enthusiasm, to a packed audience dressed in dinner jackets and formal evening wear, he stripped to the waist and showed the fascinated audience what could be seen inside the abdomen with this form of imaging. One of the most important of the applications, and the earliest developed, was imaging of the unborn baby, as ultrasound could be used to assess the size and growth of foetus to diagnose multiple pregnancy, and to give early warning of foetal abnormalities and placenta praevia. Some radiological examinations of the abdomen were no longer needed as ultrasound could be used to see both the internal dimensions of organs and their structure. This applied particularly but not only to the biliary system, where examinations such as cholecystography were no longer performed and the student's clinical experience had to be changed, decreasing the numbers of examinations for the biliary system and eliminating obstetric radiography, leading to changes in the diagnostic students' log books. Doppler ultrasound could detect blood flow and reduced the use of some contrast media studies such as arteriography and venography.

Medical ultrasound is also different from many other forms of medical imaging in that the operation of the equipment and interpretation of the findings is highly operator dependent. From the outset sonographers (radiographers or other suitably qualified health care professionals undertaking ultrasound examinations) carrying out obstetric scans reported on their findings, combining opinion gained from what they saw on the screen with the images they had taken. But difficulties were created for sonographers if they carried out abdominal scans, as many radiologists felt that technological staff without medical training should not be reporting on images and yet they were the ones carrying out the procedure. So the practice for general ultrasound examinations varied from hospital to hospital with sonographers being given differing degrees of responsibility on the reporting of their findings depending on where they worked and the attitude of the radiologists.

The first unit available to hospitals in the UK was the Diasonograph, designed and manufactured in Scotland, weighing one ton and was nicknamed the 'dinosaurograph'. In the early 1970s many hospitals in the UK were installing diagnostic ultrasound units. Dr William (Bill) Lees had started doing research into ultrasound when he worked in the physics department at The Middlesex. He was a qualified medical doctor but not a radiologist. He effectively developed an obstetric service with the help of a registered nurse, Judy Adams, both of them very respected in the ultrasound world. Dr (now Professor) William Lees took the Membership of the Royal College of Radiologists (MRCR) and opened the Ultrasound department at The Middlesex Hospital in 1974 in the basement of the X-ray department. In 1990, with the increase of ultrasound imaging demanded by clinicians, the department moved into a new department in the basement next to the Magnetic Resonance Imaging (MRI) scanners. This new department had six ultrasound bays equipped with all the modern high-tech machinery; however all obstetric scanning was carried out at University College Hospital. Two of the bays were used by radiographers carrying out gynaecological ultrasound but at The Middlesex they were not allowed to do abdominal scanning, this remaining the realm of the radiologist. Those radiographers training in ultrasound who needed to fulfil a log book requirement of

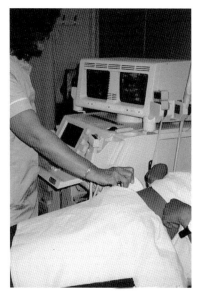

Image 42: An ultrasound examination

carrying out abdominal examinations had to be seconded to other hospitals to gain the relevant experience. For pre-diploma students the difficulties of fulfilling syllabus requirements were similar to those of the staff at The Middlesex and much the same solutions had to be found, with secondment to other centres. Naturally the theory of ultrasound had to be added to the qualification diploma syllabus which was becoming larger and larger.

It had became clear that post diploma training in Medical Ultrasound was necessary and in 1976 the Society of Radiographers registered the first students for a course of training in this specialism, a pilot course being run at the Schools of Radiography at The Middlesex. Applicants were eligible to register for the course if they had at least one year's experience in scanning and the length of the theoretical course was just over six months. There were 25-30 registrants from London and the South East and Marilyn Swann was in charge as co-ordinator and Teacher Principal (she was already co-ordinating the Nuclear Medicine course). She had done no ultrasound herself, but the set-up and the facilities at the School lent themselves to her organising the course and co-ordinating the lecture programme. The physics component was taught by staff from the Medical Physics department and very senior and experienced clinicians from around the country lectured on the techniques used. In 1977 the first examination for the Diploma in Medical Ultrasound (DMU) was held. The Middlesex School was one of the London centres offering the course in each of the following years until the Diploma ceased to be examined in 1997. The course was highly successful although there were always problems obtaining sufficient clinical experience for the students, not only for Middlesex radiographers but also for the international students, from whom there was a huge demand; even paying a fee for providing placement experience did not help with the situation as the departments were too busy. Following Marilyn's retirement in 1977 a series of tutors took responsibility for the ultrasound course. Initially Julia Lovell, Principal of the Radionuclide Imaging Course, fulfilled the role, then, when she retired (1985), Mary Lovegrove (Phillips) took over, though when she left in 1988, that year's course had to be cancelled, because of lack of qualified staff. Finally Jennifer Edie qualified in ultrasound in September, 1988 and immediately took on responsibility for the course, continuing to the School's closure.

Diagnostic Radiography

In the Diagnostic field one of the first developments of importance was the improvement of the design of the x-ray tube. Even in 1897 the January issue of *Nature* illustrated thirty two different types of tube. The basic method of producing x-rays today is essentially the same as that initially used by Roentgen in 1895. Electrons freed from a metal cathode are accelerated to a high velocity and then suddenly stopped by striking a dense, high atomic number target. However, since 1896 there have been many changes in x-ray tube design and in the means of accelerating its electrons. The early tubes all had stationary anodes, and the ability to use a short exposure in order to 'stop' the blur caused by heart beat, lung movement, or just the inability of the patient to hold still for a long exposure, was severely limited by the inability of the target to withstand the heat generated or to dissipate that heat quickly enough. The anode could become white hot when in use and the target area could melt. In addition the electronic prevention of exposure due to overheating of the tube was not then possible and the radiographer and the radiography student had to be able to understand the problems and read quite complicated cooling charts to be able to calculate allowed exposures. This necessitated a technical knowledge of the design of x-ray tubes which some radiologists thought quite unnecessary, but

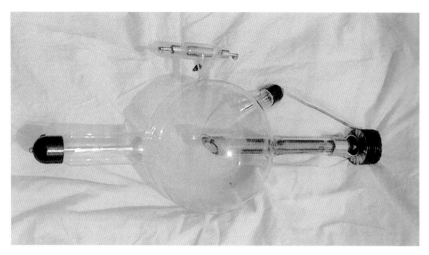

Image 43: An early x-ray tube

which was defended by the engineers who knew what damage could be caused and what it would cost to repair.

The early tubes were not designed to absorb radiation in unwanted directions, which led to a high dosage to staff, nor were the tubes electrically shock proof which meant that the users (radiologists, radiographers and students) had to understand electricity and its ability to injure or kill, and radiation and its ability to cause damage.

The major development in x-ray tube design permitting higher tube currents which allowed shorter exposures was the rotating anode. The anode would rotate at 3,600 revolutions per minute (and nowadays even higher) and was much more expensive to manufacture, costing a minimum of £600 (£9150) in 1960. The rotating anode x-ray tube allowed the electron beam to interact with a much larger target area, so that the heating of the anode was not confined to one small spot as in a stationary anode tube. The heating capacity for shorter exposures increased with the speed of rotation of the anodes but overheating was still possible and the stationary anode tube was still used on mobile and dental machines and in mammography in the 1970s, meaning that the syllabus for radiography students still had to include all the older technology as well as the new.

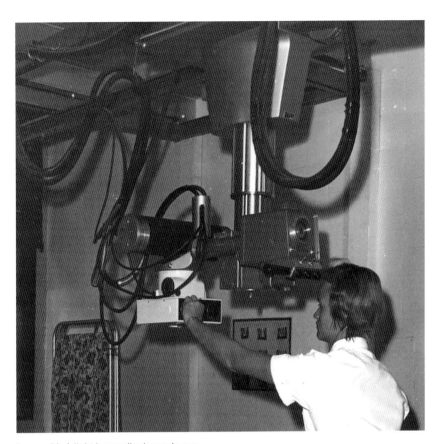

Image 44: A light beam diaphagm in use

The early images not only suffered from movement blur but also from scattered radiation generated by the body, which caused an overall fogging of the image. Scatter is radiation not of the image forming beam but, produced by interactions within the body which decreases the image contrast and definition. To reduce this, radiographers and radiologists initially used a variety of diaphragms, cones, and filters between the x-ray tube and the patient and later added grids between the patient and the x-ray film. Finally in 1921 the Potter-Bucky grid was marketed by the General Electric Company. This was designed by two radiologists, Dr Hollis Potter and Dr Gustave Bucky. Initially it was stationary and the image of the grid could be seen on the film. Subsequently it moved, then its image was not seen and it was able to remove more than 80% of the secondary radiation. Its acceptance was immediate. However it did lead to higher exposures, and

94

initially the radiographer had to remember to set and release it, as this was not done automatically.

Another technical innovation to reduce scatter and increase image quality was the use of the cone. K.C. Clark's first edition book *Positioning in Radiography* clearly demonstrated the use of round cones with the majority of illustrations having circular images showing clearly that the field of x-rays was limited by the cone. Cones were made of a lead steel combination and slid onto a retaining slot on the bottom of the x-ray tube window. They were quite long and could be brought down to actually touch the patient if a really good image was required. But this meant that the radiographer had to be absolutely sure of the relationship between an organ at depth and the surface of the patients who came in a variety of shapes, sizes and body weights. Centring of the x-ray beam was done by use of a plumb line, something which would be laughed at now. Surface Anatomy formed a large part of the technique syllabus for radiography students. These cones were replaced in the 1960s by a lead diaphragm, which incorporated a centring light, the leaves of which could be adjusted to produce any rectangular shape. Students were strongly encouraged to ensure that cone marks (clear unexposed areas) appeared on every film, to prove that the quality of the image was optimum and also to prove that the scattered radiation dose delivered to the patient was as small as possible. Because the light beam diaphragm was significantly shorter than most cones in use the number of bumps on the head that student radiographers received from positioning the patient was considerably reduced.

A further development which occurred in the 1960s was the floating top x-ray table. Before the Health and Safety laws were applied it was routine for radiographers to perform physical feats of lifting and moving heavy patients that would horrify those performing best practice nowadays. Initially positioning the patient, of whatever size, from the patient's perspective consisted of sitting at or lying on a very hard table and being asked to maintain an uncomfortable position for an unreasonable time, often while they were in pain. The patient had to be manhandled into the required position very accurately, certainly to within a centimetre. This evolved into placing a plastic covered foam mattress (2.5cm. thick) covered with a sheet on the table that allowed a degree of pushing and sliding without the patient having to move so much. The development of movable table tops, some of them four way floating, with the tube and film holder permanently aligned, allowed for much easier, more accurate and rapid positioning of the patient and certainly far less back strain and damage to staff.

Fluoroscopy is the imaging of the soft tissue systems of the body such as the gastro-intestinal tract. Initially this was done by the x-ray tube producing a low level of radiation over a long period, which then collided with a fluorescent screen shielded by a sheet of lead glass, and the image so formed was viewed directly by the radiologist. If it was the gastro-intestinal tract, the patient would swallow a radio-opaque material such as barium sulphate, or it might be inserted via an enema in the rectum. The images were faint, and to improve the view these examinations were carried out in total darkness. Radiologists would be seen walking the department for a minimum of twenty minutes in red goggles to help adjust their eyes to the dark prior to screening. During this time they could not report films, as it would ruin their dark adaptation and although not a waste of time, it was expensive. Radiographers and students had to help and reassure the patient, ensure that the equipment was properly set up in the dark, change the films and get them processed, and initially when they had not adapted to the low light level, stumble about bumping into people or equipment.

The image intensifier changed all this. In 1952 for the first time Westinghouse Inc. of the United States marketed an image intensifier which was rated at 200 times brightness gain, but the field of view was very limited at five inches circular diameter, which made it quite difficult to follow a bolus of barium down the oesophagus. These early systems were mechanically fixed to the front of the original fluorescent screens and large and bulky cameras and image intensifiers produced a grainy image on television monitors that could be seen both by the radiologist and staff and students. Over the years the size of the equipment reduced considerably whilst the quality of the image vastly improved. Dark adaption was unnecessary and examinations could be carried out in normal or in only slightly reduced lighting.

An example of the change brought about by the advent of a mobile image intensifier is its application to hip pinning. This was previously done in the operating theatre with one or two mobile stationary x-ray machines and a film holder. It was an arduous and time-consuming procedure. The mobile units had to be cleaned and moved from whichever ward they were on to theatre, covered in sterile drapes then and there were long intervals between exposures whilst the surgeon operated. The films were often wet processed, with the cassettes having to be carried by a running student to wherever the processing unit was, often in the department some distance away. There would be at least four pairs of images taken (antero-posterior and lateral) and the operation would take a minimum of two hours and often much longer, a substantial part of this time being taken up with waiting for the processing of the films. The development of the mobile "C" arm image intensifier unit which was based in theatre and could therefore be kept clean, could screen (fluoroscope) the procedure and allow an instant view, and the surgeon a much better assessment of progress. Films were often taken only at the end to prove a good result had been obtained. The time the patient was anaesthetised was significantly reduced. However, the use of the mobile image intensifier produced a number of problems. It was so easy to use that some operating theatre staff were sometimes found to have used it illegally without a radiographer being present. They had little knowledge of radiation safety, of the need to ensure that members of staff were not in the x-ray beam, nor that the x-ray tube if switched on for too long could overheat. Protocols had to be devised and obeyed with the radiographer in charge of the fluoroscopy and the imaging. Students had to be trained for this very responsible and senior role which some orthopaedic surgeons found unjustified and threatening to their rights. In some case it caused friction but dosages did come down and with common sense applied the rules were finally accepted.

Alongside developments in x-ray equipment came those in processing

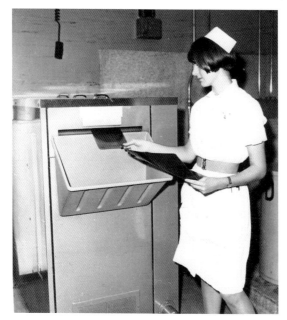

Image 45: Kodak M3 processor

of the films. In the 1950s medical x-ray films still had to be hand-processed in a succession of chemical baths, washed in running water and dried. The whole process could take a couple of hours. Image quality, reproducibility of results, and patient exposure were dependant on the user's control of processing, which was done in a photographic dark room.

The first commercial automatic processing machine was produced in 1945 in the United States and used conventional x-ray films; it could process 120 films per hour and the total cycle time for one film was about 40 mins. This was superseded in 1956 by the Kodak X-Omat processor (1956), the first roller transport processor for medical radiographs. Dry to dry time in these units was about seven minutes and The Middlesex under the guidance of Marion Frank had two of these (model M3) installed in 1962. Standing waiting for films to emerge enabled you to warm up whilst leaning on the processor and have a quick chat with colleagues. By the late 1970s high speed (ninety second) processors were installed that were much smaller and gave less time for socialising. The impact on training was that much less time was spent in the dark room by the students helping with processing, mixing chemicals and cleaning tanks, and much more time doing radiography. Automatic processors, their care, use and maintenance had to be inserted in the syllabus, whilst wet processing still had to be retained because it was used for dental films, because of their size, and in the operating theatre and for some angiography because of the need to view the images as quickly as possible.

Alongside all these developments came advances in the design of the equipment and circuitry intended to control the production of x-rays. Solid-state electronics contrasts with the earlier technologies of vacuum and gas-discharge tube and valve devices and with electro-mechanical devices (relays, switches, hard drives and other devices with moving parts). Common solid-state devices including transistors, microprocessor chips and other devices are used in computers, flash drives and more recently, solid state drives to replace mechanically rotating magnetic disc hard drives. Many more safety circuits could be inserted to protect the tube from overload and also allowed for automatic exposure devices to be used, so that the exposure automatically terminated when sufficient radiation had passed through the patient to give a good image. Penetrating power still had to be correctly selected, but the many handwritten charts of exposures required for different body parts and sizes of patients stuck above the control panel became a thing of the past. The impact of these solid state electronics was clear to the department and in the schools. Whole new areas were added to the physics and equipment syllabus as technology evolved. Transistors and computers were in and valve rectifiers were out. In the department, equipment became smaller, more complex and expensive, and local support from the on-site x-ray engineers declined in favour of a visiting engineer with oscilloscopes and circuit boards in their possession.

A number of examinations and modalities were introduced and were either successful, and stood the test of time, taking a larger and larger part in procedures, or made a brief appearance in practice and the syllabus and then were superseded and disappeared. Among the latter were examinations such as kymography, xerography, thermography and endoscopic retrograde cholangio pancreatography (ERCP). Among the former are mammography, computerised tomography, ultrasound and radionuclide imaging.

Xerography was the process of making radiographs using a metal selenium coated plate instead of a film inside a cassette. These cassettes were exposed in the normal way and the plate then processed through a xerographic processor. The resultant image was transferred to paper to produce a blue and white image. There was an edge enhancement effect in the process that highlighted differences in density in adjacent tissues. This process was in use through the mid 1970s and was used in mammographic examinations and in studies of the soft tissues of the neck. The process was brought to the department for a trial period and students were taught about the equipment. The development process was not always fool-proof and the system generally required a higher dose to achieve comparable images to conventional techniques and as a result the process had a relatively short existence as a day-to-day technique and was quickly eliminated from the syllabus. Kymography was a technique for timed exposure to enable imaging of the shape of the heart. It was already out of date in 1957 and although on the syllabus questions were never asked on the subject.

The medical use of infrared thermography started shortly after 1950 in Germany. Early infrared imaging cameras derived from military systems suffered for a long time from a poor resolution (thermal as well as spatial) and extremely high prices. Additionally there was a lack of computer hardware and software. Better

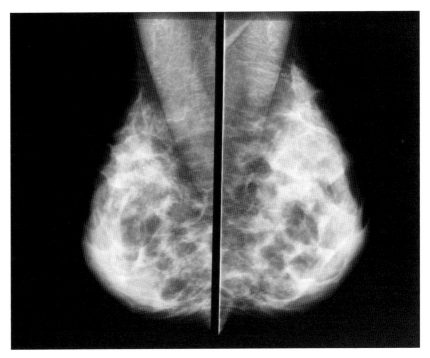

Image 46: A bilateral mammogram

technology suitable for medical purposes has been available since about 1980. John Twydle, a student from 1972 to 1974, reports that thermography was being used at The Middlesex Hospital for diagnosis of breast lesions and was performed by medical physics technicians. The procedure was not popular with the mostly female patients because the equipment in use at that time required a low ambient room temperature and one of the few places cool enough was the basement storage areas. The uninviting environment allied with the requirement of the patient to sit naked to the waist for a substantial period of time led to its unpopularity.

Mammography is the process of using low-energy-x-rays (usually around 30 kVp) to examine the human breast and is used as a diagnostic and a screening tool. The goal of the UK screening programme is the early detection of breast cancer, usually before it can be palpated, typically through detection of characteristic masses and/or micro-calcifications. It is a massive programme with all women aged between 47 and 73 years now being called for screening. Mammography is also used to aid the localisation of tumours and to help with biopsies. Although

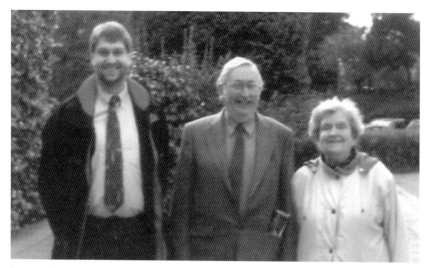

Image 47: Uwe Busch (Deputy Director of the Roentgen Museum in Germany), Godfrey Hounsfield, Marion Frank

students were taught the positioning and had to perform a certain number of mammograms prior to qualification, there is now a special programme for qualified radiographers to enable them to produce the required image in a very short time whilst still endeavouring to show care for the patient.

Endoscopic retrograde cholangio pancreatography (ERCP) was developed in 1968 and is a technique that combines the use of endoscopy and fluoroscopy to diagnose and treat certain problems of the biliary or pancreatic ductal systems. Through the endoscope, the physician can see the inside of the stomach and duodenum, and inject contrast agents into the ducts in the biliary tree and pancreas so they can be seen on x-rays. However the ability of ultrasound to image soft tissues within the abdomen without an invasive procedure has meant that imaging of the biliary tract by x-ray was rarely performed in the 1980s and the later development of non-invasive investigations such as magnetic resonance cholangio pancreatography (MRCP) has meant that ERCP is now rarely performed without therapeutic intent.

Computed tomography (CT) was developed by Godfrey Hounsfield of EMI and Dr James Ambrose, a South African radiologist working at Atkinson Morley Neuro-Surgical Hospital in London. Hounsfield was jointly awarded the Nobel Prize in

1979 for the invention. The first clinical prototype EMI scanner (Mark 1) was a brain scanner, the human body at that time being too large to fit in the aperture, and was installed in early 1972 at the Atkinson Morley Hospital, where it was used extensively to help in the diagnosis of pathology in the skull. It proved to be an immediate success and an improved version was introduced at that year's meeting of the Radiological Society of North America. Since the development of first generation CT scanners, the major technical advances include an increase of the size of aperture so that any part of the body can be imaged and to dramatically increase the speed of scanning and image reconstruction. Now 3D reconstructions are possible and CT fluoroscopy. This has been accomplished by simultaneously acquiring data through more extensive detector arrays and vastly improved computer technology. An advantage is that the images obtained can be understood by the ordinary clinician and surgeon. However there is increasing concern over the increasing use of such high radiation dose examinations for little clinical justification.

When The Middlesex Hospital acquired a CT scanner in 1978 John Twydle, who qualified at The Middlesex in 1974 and who had worked on the first whole body scanner at the Medical Research Council at Northwick Park Hospital from 1975, returned to The Middlesex to run the unit as one of the few radiographers with practical experience. The scanner had been purchased with money raised by a charity set up by a patient of the consultant radiotherapist Dr Margaret Spittle. The situation was unusual at that time with the scanner being shared between diagnostic and therapy departments. The scanner was physically located in the radiotherapy department with a mixture of patients from both departments being referred. Friday afternoons were set aside for the development of therapy planning techniques in conjunction with the images produced. Multiple slice reconstruction and an Emiplan system with 3D planning techniques were developed, linked to CT scans to ensure treatment plans matched the physical location of tumours within the body. CT enabled a number of time-consuming, highly invasive and distressing (for the patient) x-ray diagnostic examinations to be completely eliminated from the menu, including encephalography and myelography, and spelled the end of the highly skilled, time-consuming and specialised techniques required to produce images of the skull and facial bones with convention x-ray technology. CT led to much more accurate planning for radiotherapy, in which improvements continue.

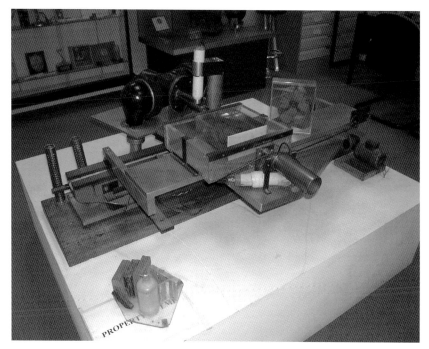

Image 48: Original lathe bed CT prototype

CT was added to the syllabus and students, both diagnostic and therapy, worked in the unit on rotation for one or two weeks at a time. Radiographic training was also given to existing staff to allow the unit to be used by on call staff if an emergency arose.

There were two further technological developments becoming important around the time of the Schools' closure. In the early days of radiography, exposure of the film was only by direct radiation and this continued for the extremities (hands and feet) well into the 1970s. For other parts of the body, as the quest for lower patient dose and more speed progressed, intensifying screens were placed inside the cassette so they sandwiched the film. Exposure of the film was achieved both by the radiation directly and by light emitted from the screens when exposed to radiation. Over the years the "speed" of the screens improved and there was a move from the well established calcium tungstate screens to "Rare Earth" screens. Film manufacturers also improved the sensitivity of emulsions in the same period achieving smaller radiation doses to the patient.

In the 1979/1980 Bunker and Herbert Hunt, from Texas in the USA, tried to corner the global market in silver and as a result silver prices rose from $11 a troy ounce to about $50 before collapsing back to $11 in 1980. Silver is a major constituent in the manufacture of film and as such film prices rose dramatically in this decade. This drove the quest towards computed radiography (CR) where film was replaced by a reusable plate. The CR plate was placed inside a cassette and exposed just as film was previously. Instead of the film being processed the CR plate was removed from the cassette inside a plate handling system and a digital image scanned from the plate. The plate was then "cleared" and replaced in the cassette ready for a new exposure. The image could be viewed electronically on a high resolution monitor or printed back onto film.

These technologies evolved into digital radiography (DR), which is a form of x-ray imaging where digital x-ray sensors are used instead of traditional film. In the last twenty years it has almost entirely taken over from conventional radiography. It has enabled the almost total elimination of chemical processing from the x-ray department which means students now spend much less time on photographic theory, and fewer staff and less space are needed for processing. The images can be previewed almost immediately for diagnostic suitability, so the patient waiting time is far less; the images are digitally stored which means much less space is required for film storage; there is less likelihood of loss or misfiling of films; and they can be transferred electronically instantaneously, which enables doctors in clinics remote from the department, off site, or indeed overseas to access and view them easily. If used properly it can significantly reduce patient radiation dose. However, when the Schools closed, the theory was known, but it was only just being put into practice, with a digital chest x-ray unit being installed at The Middlesex in 1991. Slowly the whole department became digitised and little film based technology is now used.

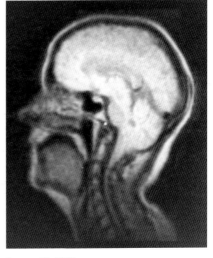

Image 49: MRI scan

The second development was Magnetic Resonance Imaging (MRI). MRI uses non-ionising radiation. It employs a powerful magnetic field, which causes the hydrogen nuclei in the water in the human body to react with radio waves having a precise resonant frequency, which further reacts with the nuclei. The result of a fairly complicated process is that photons of energy are released which can be detected by the scanner. Nuclear resonance imaging has been known to chemists since its discovery was first reported in 1946, with the first commercial Nuclear Magnetic Resonance (NMR) machines appearing in the mid-fifties and the first books on proton NMR, directed at organic chemists, being published about 1959 -1960. But the imaging of something of the size of the human body with acceptable detail in a reasonable length of time presented very large challenges and it was Sir Peter Mansfield from the University of Nottingham and Paul Lauterbur, of the University of Illinois who were finally awarded a Nobel Prize in 2003 for 'discoveries concerning magnetic resonance imaging'. MRI is a magnificent tool for showing detail within the soft tissues of the human body. It can differentiate between white and grey matter in the brain, something which a CT scanner cannot. It makes clear the anatomy of the spinal cord. It is a tremendous aid to both diagnosis and radiotherapy planning. However the first MRI scanner was not installed at The Middlesex until 1990 almost at the same time as the Schools transferred to London's City University.

Students were always taught about new developments, some of which did not survive, and others became mainstays of imaging and treatment, and if these developments were not available at The Middlesex, visits were arranged to other centres. This was often prior to their inclusion in the College of Radiographers' syllabus which took some years of gestation. In the 1980s the length of training was extended to three years and the syllabus for the Diploma of the College of Radiographers was revised to cover all these developments, with imaging for radiotherapy becoming an important component of the Principles of Radiotherapy and Oncology Syllabus (See Appendix A).

CHAPTER 4

Reaching Out

Between 1935 and 1990 more than 1200 pre and post-registration students were trained in diagnostic and/or radiotherapy radiography, medical ultrasound and nuclear medicine at The Middlesex Hospital Schools of Radiography. Many hundreds of radiographers came to the Hospital and Schools to gain valuable experience and qualifications, and to further their careers. A large number of these were from the United Kingdom but the Schools had a reputation for providing education and training for international radiographers. In the 1950s and 1960s a number of diagnostic and therapy radiologists from overseas came to The Middlesex Hospital for their radiological training, inspired by Professor Sir Brian Windeyer and Sir Harold Graham Hodgson and the reputation of the departments they had founded and developed. On returning to their own country they were usually in a position of influence either within their own teaching hospital or university, or even at Government level, and they would recommend that the technical staff should train at the same institution as themselves. Through the drive of Sir Brian and his connections with the World Health Organisation,

and the international contacts of Marion Frank, radiographers from other countries began to arrive in the early 1960s (See Appendix C). In 1966 there were twenty registered at The Middlesex Schools. Their programmes ranged from three to twelve months, covering both clinical experience and study for the Fellowship of the Society of Radiographers (FSR) and the Teachers' Endorsement (TE).

Those international radiographers who had a qualification recognised by the Radiographers Board at the CPSM were able to gain the same qualifications as UK radiographers, for example in teaching,

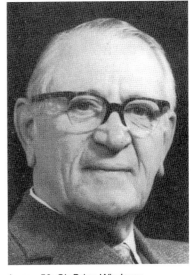

Image 50: Sir Brian Windeyer

in medical ultrasound and in radionuclide imaging (See Appendix B). This was not the case for colleagues from the Middle East and other areas where the UK qualifying diploma programme was not available. These students were able to attend relevant lecture programmes but were not eligible to sit the examinations offered by the College of Radiographers, so on successful completion of their programme these post-diploma students were given a Middlesex Hospital Schools of Radiography Certificate. This identified the programme they had attended and any success they had achieved in the internal examinations. In the 1970s and 1980s other programmes that did not specifically require the Diploma of the College of Radiographers as an entry qualification became available. Students were able to sit the Further Education Teachers' Certificate offered by various Further Education Colleges under the auspices of the City and Guilds Institute. The School of Radiography at Ipswich offered an innovative Clinical Instructors' Certificate programme as well as a Radiation Protection Supervisors' course, both of which were useful to many overseas applicants, and some shorter programmes were tailor-made for them. Many colleagues came to London for updates in modern radiographic imaging, treatment techniques, or management of a department or school of radiography and or radiotherapy. The length of

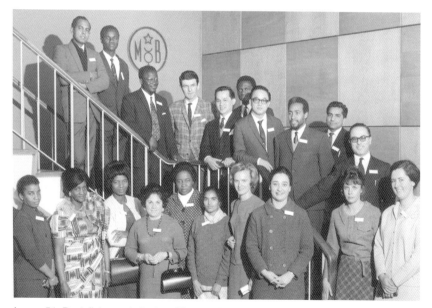

Image 51: Post diploma students at May and Baker

time they had available varied and the Schools did what they could to facilitate their requirements.

Much information has been gathered from the records of the time and from a questionnaire sent to a sample of post-diploma students and colleagues in 2008. In the questionnaire there were a few responses from radiographers who were at The Middlesex in the early 1960s but the majority came from people who had studied in the 1970s and 1980s. Post-diploma courses had been organised for some years and in 1973 The Middlesex ran the pilot Higher Diploma of the Society of Radiographers (HDSR) programme for the Society of Radiographers. Margaret McClellan, who was later to become Principal of the School of Radiography, was introduced to The Middlesex by these courses and remembers being so overawed by everything that she tried to hide by sitting behind one of the large pillars in Classroom I. It is not surprising that the Higher Diploma programmes were well attended as recognised programmes were being offered for the first time and money for overseas applicants was more easily available. This situation continued into the 1980s, but applications from overseas radiographers began to decline in the 1990s and with political instability in some areas and funds being used elsewhere, less finance was available for radiography.

Over the years a reputation was built by The Middlesex Schools of Radiography and Radiotherapy for providing top quality education and clinical experience for radiographers from other countries who then returned home to use and pass on their new-found skills. Funding for the courses and the living expenses of these radiographers came from a variety of sources. The main sponsors for the overseas radiographers not working in the UK were the World Health Organisation, the Overseas Development Agency, the Colombo Plan, the British Council and individual governments and universities. The authorities in some countries had a policy of selecting the top students in their secondary schools for radiography training and sending them to the UK without the students having any input to these decisions about their career or its development.

Countries like Australia, New Zealand, and the Republic of South Africa had a radiographic qualification recognised by the Radiographers Board at the CPSM, which enabled their radiographers to be registered in the UK. The students were therefore able to find employment at The Middlesex Hospital or elsewhere and funded their programmes from their own salaries. Additionally, in the middle 1970s teachers in Malaysia, Sri Lanka, Singapore, Hong Kong, Jamaica, Nigeria and some other African countries, who had qualified as radiographers in their own country by sitting examination papers sent out and marked by the UK Society, had later qualified as teachers in the UK. Often UK examiners would travel to undertake the viva voce examination of these students. In this way, overseas colleagues who had a recognised entry qualification for higher and specialist UK qualifications were able to sit the same examinations as their UK counterparts and gain the same recognition. UK-qualified radiographers who were also on the staff either in the departments or the Schools at The Middlesex or elsewhere in the UK attended the same courses on a day-release basis.

The majority of overseas students worked very hard, considered it a privilege to have been chosen to study in the UK, and were well aware of what was expected of them. They underwent an enormous change to their lives, suffering what can only be described as 'culture shock'. In many cases they had to adapt to a very

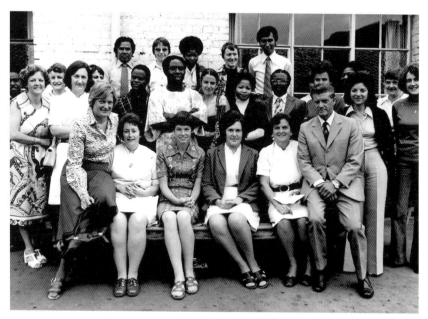

Image 52: Fourth floor roof terrace, tutors and post diploma students

different way of life, coping with an unfeeling and overcrowded London, its transport system and housing and having to study in a foreign language. In many cases, at home, they had lived in a small, supportive community close to an extended family. Most came from hot sunny countries where they spent a great deal of time outdoors, and to come to London and be confined to a small room with only one window and a view of a busy grey street must have been difficult. More personal issues revolved around leaving spouses and children behind, the high cost of living in London, being short of money, travelling into the centre on an overloaded transport system each day, or missing out on a promotion at home and the increased salary this would have given. One student was robbed on the Tube, another was worried about getting stuck in the Schools' lift, another felt that as a foreigner he needed to be 'on top of everything'. Their situation was not always appreciated by their UK counterparts, but the overall impression that emerges from responses to the questionnaire was of an ethos that was supportive, friendly, stimulating and happy, although some students found the clinical departments less welcoming than the Schools. It was clear that the support and encouragement they received helped them to overcome their difficulties and as one person said, "the worst thing was not being able to extend my stay".

The overwhelming advantages for home and overseas students were the friendships that were forged and the stimulating environment in which they found themselves. They enjoyed the inter-cultural relationships, the conferences they attended, travel in the UK and the rest of Europe, and living in London, with all it had to offer. Their best memories centred mainly on social activities with some delightful and humorous anecdotes being supplied. Chin Jin Hon, now head of radiography education in Singapore, said 'the Schools at the Middlesex had a unique personality and strength and the term global centre of post-diploma radiographic education would best describe it.'

The fourth floor of the Schools' premises at Doran House was given over to social activities for pre and post-diploma students. There was comfortable seating, a table-tennis table, a dartboard, and a piano, and outside there was a roof terrace with wooden tables and benches. There was also a kitchen used by the overseas students as somewhere to gather, chat and enjoy coffee together, although there was some argument over who was to wash up the coffee cups.

Margaret McClellan remembers two radiographers newly arrived from war-torn Uganda, anxious to know when they would have their identity cards issued as the police were sure to keep asking for them. She found it hard to reassure them. Tyrone Goh from Singapore said:

My best memory was my first meeting with Marion Frank. I flew into a cold winter in November of 1976. On arrival at Heathrow, it was so cold that I had to wear my flannel pyjamas below my suit. The pyjama pants were rather long and they showed under my suit pants. I went straight from the airport with my luggage to the School of Radiography to meet Miss Frank. At the end of the introductory meeting, Miss Frank said to me 'Chum, you must be feeling cold as I can see the pyjamas pants you are wearing underneath. In this country we have long johns used for this purpose'. True to her word, a month later, for a Christmas present, I received a pair of Marks and Spencer's long johns from Marion.

Another student remembers

Telephone calls were very expensive and I made do with airmail letters, tape-recorded messages to be sent by airmail. I was also not used to the food. At home we had rice every day and the change from our staple diet to potatoes was quite unsettling. Items like food were also expensive by our home standards and we have to save every penny to ensure that what was given by the British Council would last us through the months and have some left for travel.

At Middlesex, I learned about team working with people from different countries and their unique cultures. I did not know that it was taboo for men from Africa and the Middle East to perform chores like buying milk from the grocers, or washing up their coffee cups. They felt that it would be a disgrace to them, if their fellow countrymen or womenfolk were to hear about it. I always thought there was only one type of milk: that in powder form and in square packs, like back home. I did not know that there are so many types of fresh milk. The teachers, my fellow trainees were also an excellent lot. We could spend hours at level four (4th Floor) Middlesex drinking coffee and tea and talking about nothing.

R.P. Bhatnager, a student from India, remembers:

> *I happened to be a shy type of boy and was not used to drinking and dancing. I remember we were in a club in the Bristol countryside, everybody was dancing and enjoying themselves. I hesitated to join them and I was taken by surprise when Miss Frank pulled me in and taught me the steps of dancing. How wonderful was the moment for me one can imagine?*

'Lovely summer parties in the school, fuelled by M&S unsold food,' was a frequent memory. Tyrone Goh, from Singapore, recalls that

> *during our first Christmas, I was fostered to an English family to a place outside London. I think it was Hemel Hempstead. He was one of the managers with Kodak and they had two pretty girls aged 5 and 7. I had the best Christmas in my whole life, with turkey and pudding, followed by watching the Queen's Christmas Day message on colour TV.*

Much of this life was remembered with affection: summer parties, Christmas lunch, Teachers' Seminar Reviews, eating Greek food for the first time, visiting the Roentgen Museum in Germany and seeing the faces of students when they opened their results. One person commented on how the staff always mastered the sometimes difficult pronunciation of an overseas student's name and in doing so, made them feel welcome. They enjoyed the new imaging modalities, in-house workshops and conferences and the opening of the new premises in Foley Street. One was very proud of being asked to teach his own post-diploma colleagues. Others enjoyed the HDCR programme.

While the majority were successful in their programmes a few were not, and although they went home empty-handed, many were still appointed to positions of importance and seniority. Some of the following comments are purely anecdotal but obviously caused concern. Making a mistake in the clinical department, like not switching on the mobile unit in good time for an x-ray examination in the operating theatre and keeping the surgeon and patient under anaesthetic waiting; having to completely re-write a TDCR log-book because they had failed to maintain their anonymity; and producing a large report 'on demand' at impossibly short notice. Although they spoke English, some students found it difficult to make themselves understood to start with, as spoken English is often different from what they had been taught, and of course the English themselves have many different accents. Some memories involved failure of HDCR and how this would be received at home, difficulties with particular groups of students, and coping with the aftermath of when a DCR student was told to leave. The stress of studying for so many examinations in a short period of time, and the long hours involved in working and giving lectures for the first time all heightened their anxiety.

None of us who were there at the time will ever forget the story of Paul Draleke, who was under serious threat in Uganda from the horror of Idi Amin's regime. Marion Frank wrote a letter stating that he was due to give a key lecture at an important International Society of Radiographers' conference. This was untrue but it enabled him to cross the border and escape to the United Kingdom. He too qualified as a teacher of radiography at The Middlesex and finally emigrated to Norway, married a Norwegian, and became a senior teacher there. He used to bring a group of Norwegian students to The Middlesex annually. The first time Margaret McClellan met him, she expected a blond Norwegian and was faced with a very tall, very thin, very black Ugandan. Deliberately, no one had told her who he was.

A number of radiographers came from Singapore to take the higher professional examinations and became leaders of their field, including Karthigesu Vaithilingam and Tyrone Goh, both of whom became Presidents of the ISRRT. In the same year, 1978, Eliphas Maphosa came for three months, took and passed his Higher Diploma in the shortest time ever, and finally became Advisor in Radiography to the Government of Zimbabwe. Avis Bareki and Harriet Rickets-Ankrah became lead radiographers in their respective countries of Botswana and Ghana, and a large number of Nigerian radiographers trained as teachers at The Middlesex Schools and went on to very senior positions in their own societies. Philip Akpan, one of the first overseas students, became President of the ISRRT as well as the head of the State Registration body for Nigeria. Jemeliah Rouse, who gained her HDCR

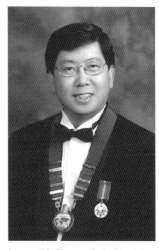

Image 53: Tyrone Goh, President of the ISRRT 2002-2006

and TDCR in Radiotherapy, became Principal of the School of Radiography in Kuala Lumpur and went on to hold a senior position at the university.

In 1983 Charles Nyabeze, a Radiotherapy Superintendent from Zimbabwe, came to The Middlesex for two years to study for the Radiotherapy HDCR and then the TDCR, but, as he was about to start the second year when he would be registered as a student teacher, he was called home. Fortunately it was agreed that he could complete most of the required hours of teaching in Zimbabwe, but would have to return to The Middlesex to cover other aspects of the syllabus. The date for his return was delayed and

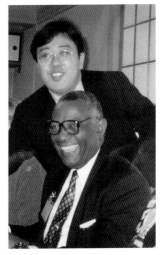

Image 54: Philip Akpan

he eventually arrived about a month before the examination, at the 'eleventh hour' as Mary Embleton, the Radiotherapy Principal, was going on leave the next day and needed to explain to Charles the last-minute teaching experiences and visits that had been arranged for him. He passed the examination.

These international students brought whole new cultural experiences, different ideas and ways of living to all those with whom they came in contact. They provided a great deal of fun, including new ideas on what constituted food, and their leaving parties were often memorable and unique. Major Mba who was seconded from the Nigerian army was awarded cardboard field marshal's epaulettes by the teaching staff at his leaving party. An Indian postgraduate student was returning home and a group of radiographers gathered very early in the morning at the West London Airport terminal in Kensington to bid him farewell. Marion Frank had armed them all with red roses to wave, which she had bought even earlier at Covent Garden. Josephat Banwha, who came from Zimbabwe, particularly remembered his sending off party. Joe had a special place in the hearts of the staff at that time, as he was a hard-working teacher for more than two years. He gelled well with the male teachers, being a supporter of Manchester United football team, and was delighted to go to one of their matches with Stuart MacKay. In Zimbabwe, Josephat was a prince in his tribe. He had already taught us a greeting in Swahili for when his wife visited, and we felt he deserved a special send-off. One of the staff got hold off a large black car, and Joe sat in the back together with his 'bodyguards'. Stuart Mackay drove, wearing a chauffeur's cap and David Chapman-Jones and Peter Hogg were the guards, all wearing black sunglasses. The female staff had to make their way to Heathrow by public transport! Once there, Joe was ushered from the car through to the departure lounge by the deferential guards and teaching staff. It was a fond farewell to a popular member of the team.

It is not surprising that the main influences in the lives of the overseas students were stated to be Marion Frank and the other members of staff. Bill Stripp, the Superintendent at the Royal National Orthopaedic Hospital, always a great supporter and teacher to students at all levels, was also frequently mentioned.

All overseas radiographers returned home, and most went on to become leaders in either their departments or other educational facilities. Several took an active part in their professional organisations as well as the International Society of Radiographers and Radiological Technicians (ISRRT), some taking high office in those organisations. A couple left the profession for family reasons, some went to work in other countries. Their time at The Middlesex enabled them to develop various training programmes in their home countries and to continue with their own education. Several became consultants and examiners to other institutions in their own lands. Many commented that their confidence had increased and they were able to speak in public and to give papers at national and international conferences. Sadly, a few returned to war-devastated countries, enormous political unrest and civil disobedience and did not survive.

In some cases the networking so engendered led to requests for help and invitations to visit the country. Marion Frank was unselfish with regard to these invitations and did not hesitate to recommend other suitably experienced radiographers to make the visit on her behalf. In 1980 Margaret McClellan visited Zimbabwe and Zambia with Marion to be trained in how to approach such visits and then in 1982 to Sudan to advise on radiography education. Such trips were not holidays. They were in Zambia for two weeks firstly to conduct the examinations and secondly to set up and deliver the lectures for a three day seminar. The visit to Sudan involved moderation of students' written work and papers for their final examinations, conducting vivas, giving lectures, visiting

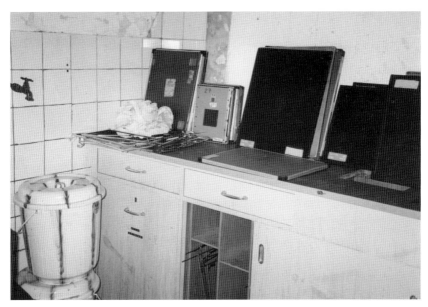

Image 55: The cassette loading area in a Gambian hospital, 2000

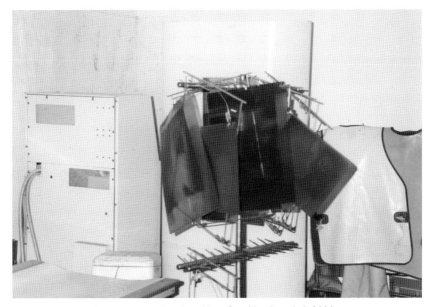

Image 56: Drying films processed by hand in a Gambian hospital, 2000

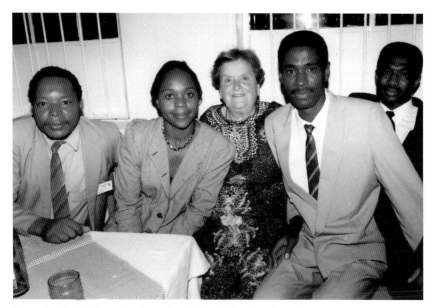

Image 57: Socialising at an ISRRT workshop in Arusha, Tanzania

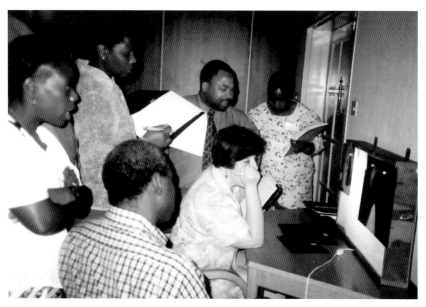

Image 58: Teaching at an ISRRT workshop, South Africa

departments and producing a written report on the training centre. In 2000 following a direct request to Marion by a local radiographic worker, Jean Harvey went to the Gambia twice. The stated objectives were to find out the current level of radiographic service, to identify any needs for service improvement, to make recommendations for future development of the service and to prioritise the recommendations for future action. Although the x-ray equipment was relatively up to date, the processing conditions were poor. The follow-up visit a year later was disappointing because very little action had been taken but Jean says she did not find this surprising because the priorities for their health care were in the treatment of patients with TB, HIV and AIDS.

Of the UK radiographers who came under the influence of the Schools, it was said by various people on numerous occasions that the schools of radiography in London and the Home Counties were like a chessboard to Marion Frank, and she would already be planning in which school her next newly-qualified radiography teacher would be placed, before they had even taken their final examination. Indeed, according to Michael Jordan, General Secretary of the Society and College of Radiographers at the time, a senior superintendent said, "Marion, the Middlesex School is all very well, but it does metastasise so". This was certainly true in the 1960s and 1970s. During that time there were thirteen schools of radiography and radiotherapy in the London area north of the River Thames. In the west they were at Central Middlesex and Hammersmith Hospitals. To the east it was Chelmsford and Southend Hospitals, and centrally they were clustered at The Middlesex, University College, the Royal Free, the Royal London, St. Bartholomew's, Westminster, and the Royal Northern Hospitals. St George's Hospital did not rebuild and move to south of the River Thames until 1980, so that was also included. Further north there was a school at Luton and Dunstable Hospital and further west at Oxford.

South of the river the schools of radiography and/or radiotherapy were to be found at St.Thomas', Guy's, King's College, Kingston, Greenwich, Guildford and the Royal Marsden Hospitals, and from 1980, St. George's Hospital and the Army school, which later became the Joint Services School at Woolwich. Of these, the Guy's and King's College schools were the largest and most active. Further out to the south and east there were schools of radiography at Bromley and Canterbury. Many of these schools were founded not only to add lustre to a hospital, but for the more mundane reason of ensuring they had a ready supply of qualified radiographers trained to their own ways.

Marion Frank's chess game was played largely north of the River Thames. At Westminster School of Radiography alone there was a succession of four Principal Teachers, three of whom had trained at The Middlesex both as students and then as teachers: Adrienne Finch (Bennett), Helen Gough, and Julia Henderson (Dodsworth). Jenny Davidson (Richmond) had the temerity to undertake radiography training at Guy's Hospital before enrolling at The Middlesex School to train as a teacher before becoming Principal at Westminster.

In the 1970s to early 1980s many of the schools in Central and West London had Principals and other teaching staff from The Middlesex. Adrienne Finch was at Central Middlesex with Pat Goodchild as Deputy, and Vivian Pearce (diagnostic) and Janet High (radiotherapy) at The Hammersmith; Margaret McClellan was first at St. Bartholomew's, and then at The Middlesex and University College Hospital on Marion Frank's retirement. Pamela Snape was at The Royal London, Hilary Weller, Olive Deaville and later Barbara Turner (from 1985) were on the staff of the school at Luton and Dunstable. Whilst in Radiotherapy Mary Embleton had also returned to The Middlesex as Principal in 1980. Only The Royal Free and Royal Northern/ Whittington Hospitals remained untouched. Even south of the River Thames was affected. Margaret Howard qualified in both diagnostic radiography and radiotherapy at The Middlesex, gaining the Fellowship examination in both modalities. She went on to be Superintendent at Guy's Hospital, later Principal of the School and going on to head the Division of Radiography at South Bank University. Mary Lovegrove (Phillips) became a Senior Teacher at King's College Hospital and followed Margaret Howard at South Bank when she retired.

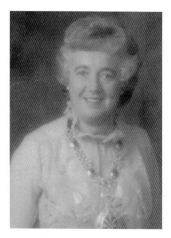

Several radiographers who went on to manage schools and departments elsewhere in the country came to The Middlesex for a period of time to gain further experience and qualifications.

Image 59: Christine Soutter President of the Society and College of Radiographers 1982/3

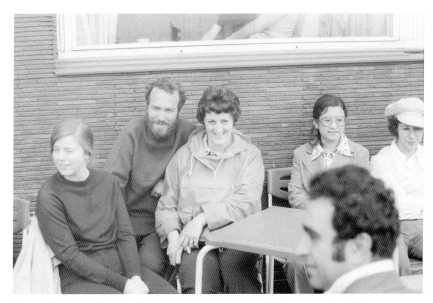

Image 60: Donald Graham (2nd left) with others on a Middlesex organised trip

Donald Graham made the furthest UK journey: seconded from Aberdeen, he gained the TDCR and returned to the Robert Gordon University as the Head of the Radiography School. Christine Soutter also qualified and gained the Fellowship examination in both modalities and in 1969 went to Manchester to run the internationally famous radiotherapy department at the Christie Hospital and Holt Radium Institute. She was later elected to the Council of the Society and College of Radiographers, becoming its President in 1982. Among others, Marjorie Moyle became the Superintendent Radiographer at Hammersmith Hospital Radiotherapy department, and Evelyn Tyrer was Principal at Kingston Hospital in the 1970s, having previously worked at the Groote Schuur Hospital in Cape Town, South Africa. Bob Bryan, seconded from Addenbrooke's Hospital as a trainee teacher, returned to Cambridge to take up the Principal's post, and Susanne Forrest (Fairbrother), became Superintendent Radiographer at King's College Hospital.

In 1966 Ann Paris, a Senior Teacher at The Middlesex School, was seconded for 'ten months' to the school at Glasgow Royal Infirmary, to rescue it when the Principal retired. The job entailed rather more than she had bargained for, because the fifty or so students had gone to ground in their original hospital departments, and Ann and a Scottish colleague, Helen Cousland, had to tour the

120

south of Scotland to round them all up. Many of their hospitals, they discovered, were situated adjacent to the local graveyards; 'Was this planned?' Ann wonders. She returned to The Middlesex clinical department as a Superintendent in charge of the neurological x-ray room and in 1969, went as Superintendent Radiographer to found the x-ray department at Northwick Park Hospital, Harrow, where she stayed until her retirement in 1997. In the early 1980s Christine Gill (Musson) became Superintendent of the x-ray department at Westminster Hospital.

There is no record of who within the Schools became examiners for the College of Radiographers, or who served on the many branch committees and working parties, but no sooner had students finished their examinations than Marion had them 'volunteering' for some extra work. Adrienne Finch remembers thinking that having successfully completed her Fellowship and Teaching Examinations, and having recently got married, that she would quietly take a back seat. Marion immediately put her up as examiner for both the qualification (MSR) and the Higher Diploma examination (HDSR), had her marking for the Rapid Results College, and within a year had her apply for the Principal's post at Westminster Hospital. Her experience was little different from anybody else's. Julia Lovell was appointed to the Education Committee of the College of Radiographers to represent Nuclear Medicine and Ultrasound. There were committees to sit on, Council members for the College and Society were needed, examiners required, working parties being set up. With Marion there was no such thing as sitting with your feet up. If 'No' was not said to her in a very definite way and with a reasonable excuse, Marion considered you had agreed. It was hard work all the way.

The College knew it could count on The Middlesex Schools in a crisis. Mary Embleton remembers that on the day of the College viva voce examinations, not long after her appointment as Principal, receiving a phone call from Veronica Atherton, Education Officer at the College. There had been a train derailment at Grantham affecting one of the examiners; please could Mary stand in until she arrived. When Mary responded that she was not an examiner the reply was "you are now!" So she grabbed some radiotherapy objects to ask the candidates questions about and rushed round to the examination hall in Queen Square. A similar incident occurred on the morning following the great storm of 1987, when both Mary and Jennifer Edie had managed to get into The Middlesex and found themselves spending the day viva examining for the College.

Two of the last teachers to qualify through The Middlesex system, Peter Hogg and Stuart MacKay, both became Professors in Radiography at Salford University. Peter became the head of the Department and for a time he was the Editor-in-Chief of the professional magazine, *Synergy*. One of the first teachers at the School, June Penney (Legg), as early as 1976, became an Associate Professor in the Department of Anatomy, and a full Professor in the Faculty of Medicine at Dalhousie University, Halifax, Nova Scotia, in the days when radiographers rarely entered academia, and certainly did not reach professorial rank. She set up a two-year training programme for American x-ray technicians at Massachusetts General Hospital in Boston, USA, and repeated this at the North Eastern Medical Centre, also in Boston. She also took an x-ray image of a sword-swallower at work, proving that he did actually swallow the sword. Jennifer Edie became Deputy Dean at the School of Community & Health Sciences, at City University, London and Mary Lovegrove became Professor in Radiography at South Bank University. Pam Berridge (Tuck), a radiotherapy teacher, became Director of Radiography Education at Cranfield University, Shrivenham. Two radiotherapy teachers wrote books that became standard texts for students and radiographers: Judy Taylor wrote *Imaging in Radiotherapy*, published by Routledge in 1988, and Pam Cherry co-wrote *Practical Radiotherapy – Physics and Equipment* (Greenwich Medical Media, 1998).

Margaret McClellan, who was nationally elected to the Council of the Society and College of Radiographers from 1984 to 1991, became Chair of its Education and Training Committee from 1988 to 1990, and was subsequently, from 1995 to 2002, elected to the Radiographers Board for Council of the Professions Supplementary to Medicine (CPSM), which was later to become the Health Professions Council (HPC). She also chaired the radiography committee setting up the breast screening programme. Adrienne Finch (Bennett) always felt that her best contribution to radiography education was to take the misunderstanding and fear out of physics at both qualification and Higher Diploma level. She became a principal lecturer at the University of Hertfordshire and Director of Education for the European and African region of the ISRRT in 1992, leading three workshops in Africa over eleven years. In 1997 she was awarded the Silver Medal of the College and Society of Radiographers, primarily for her co-ordination of the first clinical assessment scheme to be instituted by the majority of Schools of Radiography in the United Kingdom.

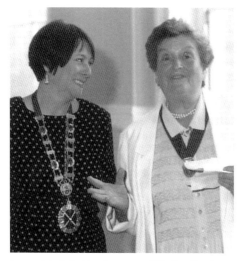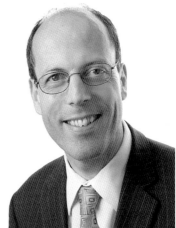

Image 61: Julia Henderson and Marion Frank   Image 62: Richard Evans

Five teachers and one former student from the School became Presidents of the College and Society of Radiographers: Mary Craig, Marion Frank, Audrey Nanette (Nan) Plowman, Christine Soutter, Olive Deaville, and Julia Henderson. This role was very demanding of time, emotion and commitment, and was the culmination of a long period of service in a variety of very responsible roles in the Society and College. In the early days, the hospital was extremely supportive of their employees' taking on these senior positions, as it was felt that it added lustre to the name of the hospital. In some cases a deputy was temporarily promoted to fulfil their role. Latterly employers were much keener to ensure that they got value for money and were not so supportive. Richard Evans began training as a diagnostic radiographer at The Middlesex School in September 1980. After working in the South of England for several years he rose to prominence in 2004, taking on the role of Chief Executive of The Society of Radiographers.

A number of those who trained at The Middlesex became significant in fields outside the immediate profession. These included Jeremy Nettle, who in 2004 was elected as the 744th Mayor of Salisbury UK, while fulfilling a demanding role in industry, and John Twydle, who was in charge of the first clinical computerised tomography scanner (CT) at Northwick Park Hospital, and is now a Senior Manager at GE Measurement and Control Systems. A number of past students and staff went into industry, including Christopher Wright, who became a business development manager for Siemens Healthcare, after having worked for Kodak in a number of roles, and Duncan Hynd, who set up his own radiotherapy equipment firm, Duncan Hynd Associates. Of those from overseas, mention must be made of Margaret Lobo, an international student from Kenya, who in 1969 completed her higher professional qualifications in a very short time; she emigrated to Australia, and became President of Soroptimist International in August 2007 for two years. In 2010 she was awarded the Order of Australia in the Queen's birthday honours list for "for service as an advocate and promoter of the status and health of women, particularly through Soroptimist International".

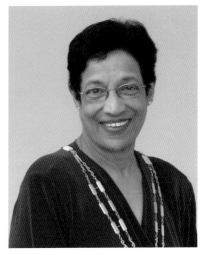

Image 63: Margaret Lobo, President of Soroptimist International, 2008

In all, more than 1000 people undertook pre-diploma courses in either diagnosis or therapy, most coming from the UK or Eire, with a few from developing countries, (See Appendix C) More than five hundred radiographers came from countries outside the UK, following a variety of programmes. The records do not show the exact numbers of UK-based radiographers who followed programmes leading to the Higher Diploma of College of Radiographers, the Diploma in Medical Ultrasound and the Diploma in Nuclear Medicine. These programmes were offered from the mid 1970s until the schools closed in 1990, and with regular annual intakes of about fifteen to each programme the total number will be more than a thousand. It is hard to put into words one's feelings at being involved in such an establishment as The Middlesex Schools of Radiography and Radiotherapy.

CHAPTER 5

Two characters who shaped The Middlesex Schools

Lucy Mary Craig OBE & Marion Frank OBE

In radiography, as in many walks of life, there are characters, possibly a little eccentric, who set the world around them 'on fire'. The Middlesex was fortunate indeed to have two such people working there at the same time and they gave the Schools their reputation and ethos. Blandness and mediocrity were not in their make-up. It is a mark of their standing in the profession and society generally, that they are still remembered with esteem, reverence and love. They were entirely different in background, education and personality, and yet they worked together to produce schools that were, according to Michael Jordan, the General Secretary of the Society and College of Radiographers during the latter half of Marion's career, 'the most prestigious in the land', their influence being spread throughout the world.

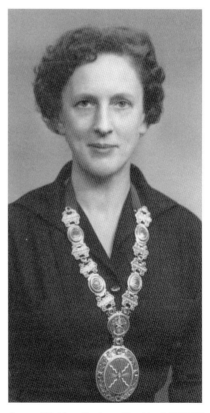

Mary's connection with The Middlesex began in 1934 and lasted until her retirement forty years later in November 1974. She was in charge of the Meyerstein Institute of Radiotherapy and Tutor to the radiotherapy students when Marion Frank was appointed Superintendent and Tutor of the Radiography Department in 1949, and the two women worked closely together in the development of the disciplines.

Lucy Mary Craig (always known as Mary) was born on 27 November 1914 in Carshalton, Surrey, the youngest of

Image 64: Mary Craig as President 1957/58

125

the four children of William and Fanny Craig. She was brought up in Carshalton and Wallington and educated at Croydon High School for Girls, where she made lifelong friends. She began her nurse education at the Norfolk & Norwich Hospital where her brother, who had been a medical student at The Middlesex Hospital, was a House Officer. Mary was not happy in the more rural environment and returned to London where she joined The Middlesex Hospital Preliminary Nurse Training School in December 1934. During her training she was greatly affected by the plight of patients with cancer, so when she qualified as a nurse, she was determined to help those patients, and joined the hospital's School of Radiography, as a student radiographer. The training in those days was in both disciplines, diagnosis and therapy. Her first appointment as a nurse and qualified radiographer was to the Collins X-ray Department, but this was only for a brief period, as she transferred to the Meyerstein Institute of Radiotherapy in December 1940. In August 1942 she accepted the position of Sister-in-Charge, but she had to give up actually treating patients a few months later because of a low blood count caused by exposure to radiation. She became Superintendent Tutor for the radiotherapy students as well as Head of Department.

The School of Radiotherapy separated from the Diagnostic School in 1949, the year in which Marion Frank was appointed as Superintendent Tutor to the X-ray Department, when the Society of Radiographers decreed that the qualifications should be divided. Despite many difficulties the diagnostic and radiotherapy education continued to be run in close co-operation until the Schools closed in 1990, primarily because Mary and Marion worked well together and were determined that the Schools and the students should remain in close partnership.

The Meyerstein Institute of Radiotherapy was created in 1936 when Dr (later to become Professor Sir) Brian Windeyer became the Medical Officer in charge. In 1942 he became the first Professor of Radiology (Therapeutic) at The Middlesex Hospital, the same year that Mary was appointed Head of Department. Thus began a very close working relationship with a mutual respect which benefited not only the Radiotherapy Department and the Schools but both the radiographic and medical staff working and training there. Sir Brian was a great supporter of the Schools, and it was as a result of his wise counsel and the respect in which he was held throughout the hospital, the university, and the medical world, that he succeeded in helping to make the Schools amongst the largest and most famous in the United Kingdom.

Throughout her life Mary Craig led by example, supporting her staff and all those who worked with her, and she was regarded throughout the Hospital as a superb head of department. Her personality and qualities of leadership instilled in all those associated with her the need for constant vigilance when using ionising radiation both for the patients' and the staff's safety. She insisted on the patient being regarded as the most important person in the hospital who should be at the centre of everyone's thoughts. She combined technical skill and professionalism with a deep understanding of the problems of the patient, their relatives, the staff and the students. Her contribution towards creating and maintaining the Department as a 'Centre of Excellence' was invaluable; working in an internationally renowned department, Mary's influence on patient care and counselling brought about changes throughout the radiotherapy world. Her professionalism did much to create and maintain the high standards of the Department which were appreciated throughout the teaching hospitals.

Mary encouraged all grades of staff to progress in their careers, many eventually taking charge of their own departments, both in the United Kingdom and abroad. She instilled in them qualities of enthusiasm, generosity in service, team spirit and meticulous care of the patients and their families. Mary worked hard both nationally and internationally for the interest of the profession; she visited departments in India and enjoyed the extensive teaching and lecturing she did at home and abroad. She was well supported by all her staff, particularly by Sister Margaret Wells, her deputy from the mid 1950s until Mary retired, when she succeeded her. On one occasion Mary was due to give a talk on 'The Art of Delegation' at a College of Radiographers' Radiotherapy Weekend Conference. She delegated Margaret Wells to do it for her. The audience regarded this as a superb example of the subject of the lecture.

For the seemingly quiet person she was Mary took on a large amount of work for the profession outside her immediate department. She stood for and was elected as a national member of the Council of The Society of Radiographers in 1948, and served until 1969. For a period of twenty one years she was regularly elected, perhaps a measure of the hard work she did and the respect in which she was held throughout the profession. She was a Vice President from 1954-1957 and President from 1957-58, the first radiotherapy radiographer and only the third woman to hold this office. She was awarded an Honorary Fellowship of The Society of Radiographers in 1959.

Her interest in education was reflected in her activities on the Council of the Society of Radiographers: she was a member of the School Inspection Panel whose role was to ensure that all recognised schools met certain minimum criteria. She was an examiner for the qualification examination (Membership of the Society of Radiographers-MSR), and a member of its Education Committee, which at that time was engaged in revising the syllabus, an enormous task. However she did not confine her interest and work to purely educational matters, she also had an interest in salaries and service, sitting for several years as a representative on Committee D of the Whitely Council, which set salary scales for radiographers in the National Health Service nationwide. Attending meetings and negotiating

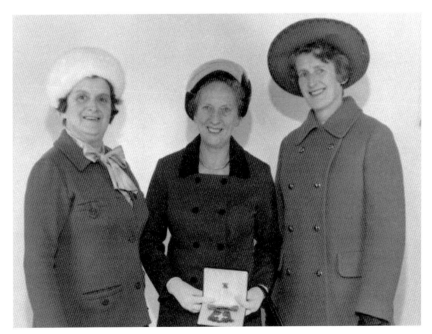

Image 65: Marion Frank, Mary Craig and Margaret Wells on the award of the OBE to Mary, 1972

salaries with officials who were determined not to allow more than the minimum salary increase and little improvement in conditions must have been difficult and draining. Obviously she strongly represented the radiotherapy interest on this body, but it was clear that she also had the general welfare and professional good standing of all radiographers at heart.

In the late 1960s Mary and her colleague Noreen Chesney were the first all-female team of School Inspectors and examiners selected by the Council of the Society of Radiographers to go overseas when they visited the Schools in Hong Kong. Nowadays nobody would think this extraordinary, but then it was primarily men from the Society who went abroad, and they felt that females might well be put at risk travelling alone to some fairly distant and to them undeveloped territories.

Mary was also a member of the Radiographers Board at the Council for Professions Supplementary to Medicine (CPSM). The CPSM was the regulatory body for all professions supplementary to medicine apart from Nursing, a role now fulfilled by the Health Professions Council (HPC). Mary served on the Board from its inception in 1962, when obviously the decisions made set precedents for the future, and thus were crucial. She was Chairman from 1970 until 1974 and was Vice-Chairman when she retired in 1974. All this unpaid work was carried out in addition to her normal workload.

As part of the Society's Golden Jubilee celebrations in 1970 Mary was one of ten radiographers who were awarded a Gold Medal, and in 1972 she was honoured by the Queen with an OBE, in well-deserved recognition of her outstanding work.

The Sir Malcolm Sargent Fund for Cancer in Children was founded in 1968 and it was a measure of the respect in which she was held and her great experience in all aspects of cancer care which made her a most suitable founder member and trustee. A fellow member was Marjorie Marriott, who had been Matron at The Middlesex Hospital (1946-1965). Mary was not pleased when the Fund changed its name to Clic Sargent in 2005, probably because she did not like the acronym and felt that it detracted from the serious aims of the fund, although CLIC was another organisation, Cancer and Leukaemia in Childhood, with very similar aims.

Mary retired in November 1974 after thirty-four years as Sister-in-Charge of the Radiotherapy Department and Principal of the School of Radiotherapy. The occasion was marked by a considerable gathering of past and present staff; a tea party was held in the afternoon in The Middlesex Hospital Board Room followed by a candlelight supper in John Astor House (the Nurses' home). It was a example of the great respect, affection and admiration with which Mary was regarded both professionally and personally that this gathering included not only past and present members of staff with whom Mary had been associated but also radiotherapists, radiographers, student radiographers, physicists, technicians, hospital domestic and trades staff, and porters. Also present were radiographers who had never worked with Mary but were there as her friends and colleagues. Her retirement gift was a new, gleaming, deep blue Austin Mini, the iconic car designed by Sir Alex Issigonis. It had been smuggled into that hallowed room, The Middlesex Hospital Boardroom, no mean feat. This was no doubt due to the great influence and organisational skills of Sir Brian Windeyer and the co-operation of the front hall porters; no one dared say 'no' to him. When the car was presented it was be-ribboned and flower bedecked. A chart had been drawn up and contributors were invited to 'buy' various parts of the car; apparently the roof was donated by the medical staff in Hong Kong. We have no record of which model this was or exactly how much it cost, but it was probably between £850 and £1000 (£8,500-£10,000 today), an enormous sum to have raised at this time and a tribute to the respect and love with which she was held. Mary had always enjoyed using the hospital car so it seemed a very suitable gift. It gave her mobility, enabling her to travel (somebody said 'trundle' - we have no idea what her driving was like) round the countryside visiting friends and relations and taking mini holidays. Professor Sir Brian Windeyer gave a tribute to Mary, full of sincerity and wit, and evidence of his high regard for all that she had done for the Meyerstein Institute and the Hospital.

Mary Craig lived in Bloomsbury, London all her working life. She had a small circle of very close friends going back to school days and her early days in nursing, but she never lost her delight in meeting and getting to know new people of all ages and backgrounds. She liked to go regularly to the theatre and concerts and she also took a great interest in local history and went often on guided walks in various areas of London. Her interests were varied: she read widely, history, biography and novels, especially the classics, and particularly French ones to preserve her

130

interest in France and the language. Her main hobbies were in the countryside, bird-watching, walking and identifying wild flowers. She enjoyed holidays at home and abroad, particularly when they were in moorlands or mountains. She adored being with her brothers Dan and Edward, and particularly enjoyed sailing with the family; its discomforts never fazed her. Once when they had sailed to France she sent a postcard to the department in which she remarked they had not had to alter the set of the sails for the entire journey. She thought this an ideal situation.

Mary never married but was dearly loved by her seven nieces and nephews, their spouses and their families, twenty great-nieces and nephews and thirty-two great-great-nieces and nephews. She remarked to one family member that when she was having difficulty sleeping she would try to remember everyone by name and their place in the family instead of counting sheep! She was a tremendous friend to all of them, always cheerful and positive, interested in everything they did, encouraging, enthusiastic, perceptive, caring, and a great support. One of Mary's nieces worked as Sir Brian's secretary for a year and had the opportunity to see the professional Mary, totally efficient, expecting high standards from her staff, at the same time being admired by everyone and loved by the patients. She noted how she wore her uniform as a Senior Sister with pride. This was quite different from the scattiness she was rather renowned for at home. When Mary went to Buckingham Palace to receive her OBE, she borrowed a handbag from a friend, and when the handbag was returned the medal was still inside. It was not unexpected and her timing was unique: she never quite missed a train although the person behind her probably did.

Mary's greatest attributes were probably her amazing ability to communicate with everyone with whom she came into contact and her sensitivity to people's needs. It was not what she asked but the manner in which she asked which made everyone feel she was caring for them as individuals. She invariably received the same positive response whether she was asking a senior manager in the administration or a member of the domestic staff. One of her nephews commented that she had an ability to state an opposing point of view, to remind one of uncomfortable truths or obligations without initiating an argument or belittling one. Words were very important to her: she had her own way of saying things. A favourite phrase with which she would dismiss some petty squabble or troublesome irritation was "I just can't be doing with that." She gave people confidence and encouraged them to take decisions themselves. She expected one to have researched those decisions carefully and said she would support you whatever the outcome, at least in public. Everyone made very sure they did not let her down.

The last seven years of Mary's life were spent in Hazeldene Retirement Home in Gosport, close to some members of her family. Life for her then was not easy, but was made better by the wonderful care she received from the staff, who were especially sensitive to her needs. She loved having regular visits from her family and longstanding friends, in particular Margaret Wells, who had worked with her most of her professional life, and was not that much younger. Margaret made the journey from Central London to Gosport on many occasions, no mean feat, particularly as she herself became increasingly fragile.

Apart from her dedication to her work, her quiet, steely determination and her strong support for her family and friends, Mary's philosophy was based on her strong Scottish Presbyterian background, her work for her church and her very strong faith, which was such a vital force. She did much to create and maintain the high standards of The Meyerstein Institute of Radiotherapy at The Middlesex. She schooled to her own standard many radiographers, and she instilled qualities of enthusiasm, generosity in service, team spirit and meticulous care of the patient. Those who knew her well remember her with great affection; she was a truly remarkable person.

Marion Frank, the second of the distinguished developers of radiography at The Middlesex Hospital deserving of special mention, was born on December 11, 1920 in Cottbus, a town in eastern Germany, politically overtaken by the Nazis and then at the end of the war by the Russians, finally in 1949 becoming part of the communist German Democratic Republic (East Germany). She died on September 15, 2011 in London, England, a country where she settled happily and of whose citizenship she was enormously proud. The stories surrounding her are legion, and there is sadly room for only a few of them to be told here.

Marion was a twin, eight minutes younger than her dearly loved sister Ellen. Although the family did not follow the Jewish tradition, their Jewish roots put them in mortal danger and they became refugees from the Nazi regime. The twins came to Britain aged 17, direct from a year's schooling in Switzerland, and lived for the first few months with the family of a doctor in Sussex, the father of one of their school friends, who had sponsored their entry. They were followed by their younger brother on a Kindertransport, a scheme designed to evacuate threatened children from Germany, and, later on, by their parents, who escaped thanks to professional contacts in the UK wool trade, with which the family were involved, and they went to live in Huddersfield. Their brother, when he was old enough, joined the British army and was selected to join an elite commando troop, the X troop. Tragically, he was killed at the D-Day landings, and was buried in Normandy. Marion visited his grave in Normandy at least once a year, preferably in early June.

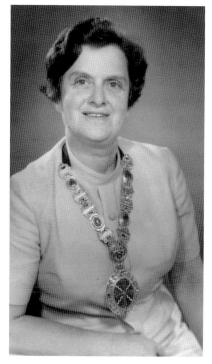

Marion wanted to study medicine but lacked both the educational certificates and the money, although she did try

Image 66: Marion Frank as President 1967/1968

later to get her first MB. So at the age of eighteen she and Ellen found jobs in the post-mortem room at London's Royal Northern Hospital. Kathleen Clark who worked at the Ilford Radiographic Department but who had retained her contacts with the Royal Northern had heard of the German twins and came to talk to them, telling them they should train as radiographers.

Six months into their training, on September 3, 1939, war was declared, and as stateless refugees (they had been stripped of their German citizenship),classified as enemy aliens, they were forbidden to work in restricted areas, such as London. Dr Stanley Scott Park, the Consultant Radiologist at the Western Infirmary, Glasgow, agreed, after interviewing them, to take them into his department to complete their training. They were then living in Huddersfield with their parents and had not enough money for the fare to Glasgow, so they walked to Leeds and paid the fare from there, a measure of their determination. They qualified

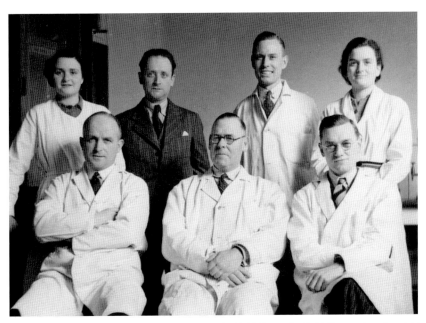

Image 67: Royal Northern Hospital Pathology Staff 1938, on the left Ellen and on the right Marion Frank

in November 1941 but finding a job with their background was difficult. They agreed to look for jobs independently, the first time the twins had been separated in twenty-one years. It took thirty-two applications before Marion was taken on at Putney Hospital in London when fear of German 'Fifth Columnists' had subsided. Ellen found a job in the mobile unit in Leicester, and later at St. Bartholomew's Hospital in London.

The war years, the rationing, the blackout and the bombing, produced many problems and challenges. One evening a dance hall near Putney Bridge was bombed; the bodies of the dead youngsters were laid out on the grass outside Putney Hospital, and Marion along with all the staff had to exercise great control when they were asked to try to identify the bodies, and when relatives arrived wanting to see their loved ones. Once she was suspected of being a spy because she was German and was seen typing up some papers in an office. Whilst on her bicycle she was stopped by the police for infringing lighting regulations and fined £20 (two and a half week's salary), addressing the magistrate as 'Your Majesty', and causing great hilarity. Caught outside during a raid she would sleep on the

Underground platform or in public air raid shelters with many hundreds of others. She accepted the crowded conditions but dreaded the crush of getting down the stairs, when people might trip and fall.

Marion was always able to focus on what she wanted to do and would brook no defeat, a trait for which many admired her but which grated with some. However her exceptional dedication, willingness to work and learn were already apparent and much appreciated, but even in those early years there were detractors who could not cope with the force of her personality. Still the staff at Putney hospital were very kind to her. When her brother died in June 1944, the Matron travelled to Huddersfield with her so she need not go alone and it was Dr Douglas Freebody, a senior orthopaedic surgeon at Putney, who signed Marion's papers when she applied for British Citizenship in 1947.

Marion was keen to become a radiography teacher, but her practical experience was limited to a two-roomed x-ray department with only one tube, without electrical shock-proofing, so she applied for a post in Derby and was appointed as a Senior Radiographer in June 1944, just after D-Day. Marion always said that it was here that she learned to be a real radiographer from the Superintendent Radiographer, George Lovell Stiles. He would ask each patient how they had received their injury, exactly where the pain was and what limitations they had; from this information he decided which projections to take. Marion took all this on board and it became an integral part of her teaching of Radiographic Technique. She ended up working as a full time teacher in the School of Radiography in Derby, and in 1947 she studied for the Fellowship of the Society of Radiographers' Examination. In those days both diagnostic radiography and radiotherapy were included in the syllabus, and her experience in radiotherapy was negligible, but she met a radiologist from The Middlesex Hospital who suggested she should study there if she wanted to learn about radiotherapy. She was accepted for three months' post-diploma experience, unpaid, starting in mid-February. At The Middlesex she met Professor Brian Windeyer, who was very impressed that she was taking leave without pay. Mary Craig was already in charge of the Department, and between radiotherapists, physicists and radiographers Marion was introduced to every aspect of radiotherapy. Winter 1947 was legendary for its length, freezing temperatures and depth of snow, and post-war rationing meant that nobody had heating so she did all her studying in bed to keep warm. She passed the Fellowship Examination (FSR) in 1947, and nine years later, in 1956, gained her Teachers' Endorsement (TE), at the first examination.

Marion wanted to broaden her experience. The USA was next on her list, but as she had no visa she travelled to Canada intending to try to get across the border from there. With her qualification papers and five pounds (£120), the maximum one could take out of the country because of currency regulations, she travelled steerage on a cargo boat from Liverpool. The journey took seventeen days and was very rough. Her father had told her that under no circumstances was she to play poker, but she enjoyed an occasional flutter and after watching the sailors play for a while she joined in. She arrived in Canada with twenty four pounds, the equivalent of £550 today.

Her first job was at the Waterloo Hospital, Kitchener, near to Toronto – which provided accommodation. In this small hospital she was expected to carry out tasks for which she was not trained, and which would not have been countenanced in the UK, for example to diagnose from the images, to treat patients with radiotherapy for the common cold, and to carry out Electrocardiograms (ECGs). She handed in her notice and, apparently with no source of income, she applied to a circus to be a human cannon ball: she finally refused to take the job as it also allegedly involved sleeping with the circus manager (the story she told to gentler souls was that the circus manager told her she was too fat, although in fact at that time she was very slim!).

Finally Marion obtained a job at the Neurological Institute in Montreal, where she said she gained great radiographic experience. It was French-speaking, which was easy for her after living in Switzerland, but wanting to save enough money to be able to return to England if she was required, she needed free accommodation. A block of flats were advertising for someone to stoke their central heating boiler at night, and she agreed to take the job if she could stay in the basement for free, with a camp bed next to the boiler and a telephone next to her bed. But one day at work, a radiologist asked her, "Why are you always so dirty when you come to work?" She explained her circumstances: there were no facilities for washing. He immediately suggested that she share a flat with his two daughters, where she was able to have a bath every day. She remained friends with one of the daughters throughout her life.

In 1948, Professor Brian Windeyer wrote to her to say that Sister Joan Parbery, Superintendent Radiographer of the X-ray Department and Principal of the School at The Middlesex was leaving, and even though Marion was not a nurse he would like her to apply for the job. Up until then the radiographers in charge of both the x-ray and radiotherapy departments at The Middlesex were qualified nurses with a radiographic qualification. He and Dr Graham Hodgson asked Marion to visit the Mayo Clinic on her way home, to see how they organised their automatic processing. She learnt a great deal, and was offered a scholarship to do research for Kodak, but she refused as she did not want to be tied to one firm. She wanted a job which she knew would give her great opportunities.

She journeyed home, worrying about the prospect of a formal interview at a big London hospital. She travelled steerage on the Queen Elizabeth and a doctor on board advised her that she needed a hat for the interview. Back in London, from the top deck of the bus she spotted what she thought was a hat shop. She found it sold lampshades, not hats, but she bought one, took out the middle, and wore it. Marion was appointed, and she and Muriel Guest, the deputy in the department, who had a mathematics degree from Oxford, became great friends; Muriel lectured to the students and taught Marion a more academic approach to study. It was perhaps a mark of her determination to succeed despite the odds against her, that ten years previously both Marion and Ellen had applied to The Middlesex to train as radiographers but were not accepted because of their German origins; now Marion was the Superintendent and Principal.

Marion started at The Middlesex in March 1949. Then it had six x-ray rooms with open high tension (voltage) valves which had to be discharged each evening. There had been little change since 1935 and modernisation was certainly required. From the beginning she was made very welcome. The deputy appointed after Muriel Guest left was Sister Stella de Grandi, whom she found very supportive; they got on extremely well and became very good friends. Mary Craig was in charge of the Radiotherapy Department, and she and Marion worked closely together. Marion learned a lot from her and found her a great influence. Kathleen Clark's Ilford's training department was at Tavistock House nearby; Kathleen visited The Middlesex quite frequently and the friendship lasted until Kathleen's death in 1968.

Marion was very keen to integrate the School and the Department. There was a structured curriculum which had been set up by Joan Parbery and Mary Craig; but no formal timetable of lectures. Students were taken out of the Department when lecturers and space were available and the departments were not busy, and this was changed to a regular timetable. Marion asked experienced departmental radiographers to lecture in Radiographic Technique, the subject in which they were the experts, and this developed their talents too. She also instituted practical experience in other specialist hospitals to increase the students' skills and make them more employable.

The Middlesex X-ray Department was one of the first to install automatic processing; Marion's knowledge gained from the Mayo Clinic was very useful. Two Kodak X-Omat processing units were purchased and installed in which x-ray films took only seven minutes to process from dry film to dry instead of the long wait for the wet, delicate and sometimes damaged films which had come out of the Department darkroom in the past. Marion also ensured that silver recovery with steel wool was used effectively; until then much of the silver from the film emulsion had gone down the drain, an expensive waste of resources and harmful for the environment.

For many years Marion was a Society of Radiographers examiner in both the written papers and viva voce (oral) in the Membership, Fellowship, Higher Diploma, Teachers' Endorsement and Diploma Examinations. In 1961 she was elected a national member of the Council of the Society of Radiographers, serving until June 1973, and she sat on several of the Standing Committees. The Education Committee was probably the one she most enjoyed, as she felt she could influence the education of radiographers both nationally and internationally; she was a co-opted member of this committee from July 1973 until June 1981. In 1965 she was elected one of the Vice-Presidents and in 1967 President of the Society of Radiographers. Always aware of her German roots, she told the Council that she would understand if they did not want her as President because of her German accent. She was elected unanimously.

Marion's Presidential year coincided with two significant events: the Society of Radiographers' move into new headquarters in Upper Wimpole Street, and the Schools' into their new premises in Foley Street. She was never one to miss an opportunity to raise money, so the informal party to celebrate the new Schools' premises was a fund-raising event for the Furniture Fund for the Society's new headquarters. In 1968 the guest invited to open the Society's Annual Conference was Brian Windeyer, Marion's acknowledgement of the important part he had played in her career and the development of the Schools at The Middlesex. The year was quite an experience for the staff in the Schools at that time and a real insight into the commitment required of a President. The number of meetings to be attended, the papers to be read, the mountain of qualifying and membership certificates to be signed, the decisions to be considered, the lectures to prepare and the travelling all over the country are just a few that immediately come to mind.

In April 1976, because of College of Radiographers' rules, Marion resigned as Superintendent of The Middlesex X-ray Department to become full time Principal of the School, a post she held until her retirement in 1981. She was invited to give the Society of Radiographers' 1975 Welbeck Memorial Lecture, and was awarded the Welbeck Memorial Medal.

As a radiography teacher Marion was famous internationally. She had always taken a keen interest in any international radiographic activities and Sir Brian Windeyer was very far sighted and internationally orientated. On their return home the overseas doctors gaining experience in the X-ray and Radiotherapy Departments would send their radiographers and students to The Middlesex for training. In 1953 Marion attended an International Congress in Copenhagen and visited departments in Stockholm and Hamburg, including St. George's Hospital, where there is a memorial for all the radiation martyrs. In 1959 the idea of an International Society was proposed at a meeting during the International Congress of Radiology in Munich. The International Society of Radiographers and Radiological Technicians (ISRRT) was officially founded in Montreal in 1962. Marion was a founder member, she said partly because she spoke German and French. Kathleen Clark, Evelyn Tyrer and Marion formulated the Education Policy of the new Society; Marion was Chairman of the Education Committee until 1977 and Vice-President (Europe and Africa) until 1973. She organised Teachers' Seminars for the International Society in London in 1966, Copenhagen in 1969, Nairobi in 1972, Kuala Lumpur in 1975, Thunder Bay, Canada, in 1978 and finally Lagos in 1980. In 1985 she was elected Regional

Chairman (Europe and Africa) of the Education Committee until this role was taken over by Susan Needham (Tinker), a past Middlesex teacher, and then by Adrienne Finch (Bennett) a past Deputy Principal of the School. Marion retained her interest and involvement in the Society even after her retirement, always willing to advise, help and support.

Marion attracted a large number of post qualification radiographers to the Schools of Radiography through her contacts, hard work and charisma. A number of the stories of her successes are given in Chapter 4, but 166 post-diploma students from fifty different counties (listed in Appendix C) were trained under Marion's tutelage, ninety two of these employed as teachers in their own countries. Not only did she look after them academically, but socially too, ensuring they saw the sights in London, including a dress rehearsal of Trooping the Colour and one of her favourites, greyhound racing at White City. She lent a Nigerian couple money to have their baby son circumcised; when they repaid her she took a group out to the cafe across the road saying "I shall treat you with my circumcision money". She loved organising theatre trips: *My Fair Lady, West Side Story, Cats, Starlight Express* were all visited by large parties under her auspices. At the Society of Radiographers' Twenty Fourth Annual Conference in London in 1970, the Society's Golden Jubilee Year, Marion extended an invitation to all overseas radiographers to attend a buffet lunch at The Middlesex Hospital; more than eighty radiographers from twenty five different countries attended. It was a joyous occasion, and an opportunity for old friends to meet, along with doyens of the profession, including past Presidents from the 1950s onwards.

Marion's involvement in the international radiographic scene was considerable; in 1969 she was made an Honorary Member of the New Zealand Society of Radiographers, and in 1977 an Honorary Member of Special Distinction of the Netherlands Society. In 1971 she was invited by the World Health Organisation (WHO) to attend a WHO and International Atomic Energy Authority meeting in Tehran to discuss the training of radiographers and other technical staff. In 1977 in Brussels and 1979 in Munich she attended WHO meetings of experts investigating the Efficacy and Efficiency of Diagnostic Applications of Radiation and Radio-nuclides, and in 1978, in Geneva, another WHO meeting, this time on Technical and Organisational Policy in Radiation Medicine. 1980 was a particularly busy year for her, attending WHO meetings twice in Munich and once in Copenhagen; the first event was a Consultation on Radiological Services, Needs and Means, the last a meeting of experts on Quality Assurance in Diagnostic Radiology.

Marion's expertise in Radiation Medicine and Radiographic Training was world renowned and in 1978 the Sudanese Minister of Health invited her to Khartoum as an Advisor under the auspices of the British Council. A year later she was invited by the Zambian Government as an Advisor; she was made an Honorary Member of the Zambian Radiological Society and in 1983 attended a

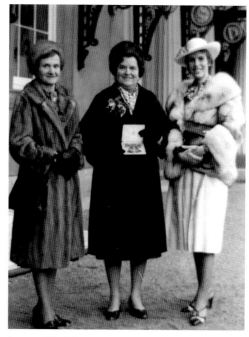

Image 68: Ellen, Marion & Jean Harvey outside Buckingham Palace, 1981

Quality Assurance Workshop in Harare. Marion was unselfish with regard to her overseas visits, and did not hesitate to recommend other radiographers to make the visit on her behalf. Both Margaret McClellan and Jean Harvey went to Africa following invitations to Marion.

Marion was also an active member of the British Institute of Radiology. In 1973, she was invited to address the Sixth Postgraduate Course in Edinburgh, her topic 'Modern Radiological Methods and the Place of the Radiographer in the X-Ray Department'. In 1980 she was made an Honorary Member of the Royal College of Radiologists, the first radiographer to be awarded such an honour. The following year, when she retired from The Middlesex, her great contribution to all things radiographic was recognised by the Queen with the award of an OBE. She attended the ceremony in the ballroom at Buckingham Palace with her sister Ellen and Jean Harvey, the Superintendent of the X-ray Department. Marion delightedly told the tale of how during her investiture the Queen asked her what she did; she proudly replied "I am a radiographer". Her wish for her retirement gift was a superb example of her generosity towards others. Anyone wishing to contribute towards her 'Gift' was invited to buy a brick for a retirement cottage which was being built in Newbury where there was a development of properties for retired Middlesex Hospital staff; more than £15,000 (about £154,000) was raised. It goes without saying that Marion's retirement party was a very jolly affair. There were strict instructions for no personal presents and there was a review featuring Marion's life presented by present radiographic staff and students with Richard Evans doing his famous impersonation of his boss.

Marion's whole life, professional and social, was mainly centred on radiography, after of course, her family. She was never happier than when organising a social gathering for just a few - or a hundred or more. She loved food, and in her early days was taken to the Ritz in Montreal by a boyfriend who suggested that she ate what she liked. She started at the top of the menu and ate her way to the bottom, astounding both her host and the waiters. Apparently once when dining with Lord and Lady Astor and being faced with an unknown dish, quail, she ate the whole bird. She said she would feel the beak going down till the day she died. Her frankfurter parties were legend and are described in Chapter 6. Schmidt's, the German restaurant in Charlotte Street, offered her a job at a significantly increased salary because she was so knowledgeable and such a good saleswoman. She turned it down.

Most of Marion's friends have a story either about her driving or her car; and it was typical that she herself laughed about her own driving exploits. Most of the experiences were harmless, but they nonetheless left an indelible impression on those who lived through them. They provided hours of amusement later on, in the retelling, and helped to cement her larger-than-life reputation. Her driving was, to put it mildly, erratic, speedy and very finely judged. She would hurtle through cobbled mews in Bayswater, across main streets, without a glance or even a hover of a foot on the brake. She burnt out clutches regularly but never had a serious accident. Marion was generous at giving lifts; it never occurred to her that she might make her passengers queasy, and she expected them to get out in the most inappropriate locations. Christine Soutter balked at getting out into the traffic on Park Lane and was dropped off at Marble Arch in the middle of the island. Another person with a suitcase, trying to reach an airport, was left on the wrong side of a German autobahn. She tipped out a very distinguished Dutch radiographer, Dien Van Dijk on the M4 leaving her to be picked up by Valerie Sharpe (Crown) whom Marion had passed at high speed and whom she had spotted was on her own. Marion's car would be lent to do complicated errands, usually carrying a non-English-speaking visitor with family and many suitcases and involving extracting the car from a jammed parking space, filling the car with petrol and checking the oil, before delivering the visitors to the airport.

Marion did not back down to officialdom; on one occasion she had parked her car in a no-go area, and when she returned she found a policeman preparing to have it towed away. She remonstrated with him, her main line of defence being that the seat was still warm so the car could not have been there that long; the car did not go to the pound. Once she arrived at British immigration with an Australian radiologist whose entry permit had run out. Not only did she get him in, she also got his permit extended for a further two years. Both the policeman and the immigration officer learnt, as had many radiographers and teachers before them, that it was impossible to say 'No' to Marion Frank.

No one will forget the familiar voice on the telephone (often at 7am), in a conversation, or a lecture, as without preamble she said, "I have just three things to say" but often continued to five or more. She refused to have a telephone answering machine: "as then I would have to return the calls". On her many trips abroad she always travelled 'cattle class', never entertained the idea of taking a taxi, and if you travelled with her you had to be prepared for some pretty basic accommodation.

From her first day at The Middlesex Marion lived in at Marlborough Court, until it closed in 1975, when she moved to a flat in nearby Lancaster Gate. She felt that Marlborough Court provided suitable safe accommodation in Central London for young adults coming to the capital for the first time, giving them the opportunity to integrate with their peers and members of the hospital staff. Fifty years later a group of past students still remember how concerned Marion was when they said they were moving out into a flat.

Marion's home very quickly became the place where colleagues and friends from all walks of life gathered; her door was always open and enough food always in

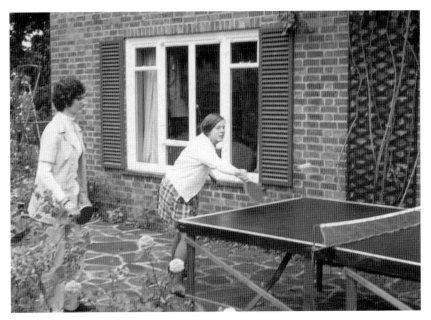

Image 69: Table tennis at a garden party at Ellen's home

the fridge. Her visitors' book contained most of the names of the 'great and the good' in the world of radiography, as well as a large number of others. She loved having people to stay and when they did they never knew who else would be there. Marion more than once commented that she was glad there were only two sexes because accommodating her overnight guests would otherwise have been so much more difficult. She was very organised: when a guest was leaving they made up the bed with clean sheets for the next visitor, putting the dirty linen in the washing machine.

In 1981, the night before the wedding of Prince Charles and Lady Diana Spencer, Marion invited family and friends to a supper party before going into Hyde Park, just across the road, to enjoy the fireworks. Her flat was packed and it appeared that most were staying. Officially there were enough beds for six people if you did not mind who you shared with and sometimes a sleeping body would be seen in the bath. That night there were at least fifteen. Margaret McClellan and a friend were guests and intended to drive home when the fireworks were over. Losing the main party in the floods of people that were good-naturedly trying to leave Hyde Park, they eventually located their car, only to find it had been blocked in and they

144

had no idea by whom. Marion found them a place to lay their weary heads – in the hallway with a cushion and a sheet, not much – but enough. Her hospitality and generosity were legendary.

Her sister, Ellen, and her family were always hospitable to Marion's friends. Once a year their garden, complete with swimming pool, was opened to a picnic party with invitations extended to staff and international students and their partners and children. There could be a hundred there, and it must have been a happy memory for many of those when they went home to a very different countryside.

Marion's final honours were awarded to her in retirement: in 1994 she was presented with an honorary MSc from South Bank University, in 1995 The Society and College of Radiographers' Gold medal in recognition of her services to radiography, in 1997 London's City University conferred on her an Honorary Doctorate of Science, and in 2010 she was given the Dien Van Dijk award of the ISRRT, for services to international radiography.

She involved herself with other organisations as well, including The Osler Club (for those interested in the history of medicine), and The Royal Surgical Aid Society, where she was one of their Vice-Presidents. The Society has four care homes for the elderly, particularly those with dementia; as part of her role Marion visited these homes regularly. For many years she was secretary of The Middlesex Hospital Twenty Five Club, for staff who had worked at the hospital for twenty five years or more, organising their social occasions. For sixteen years she was Chairman of Heron Court Co Ltd. (her home after Marlborough Court closed), where all the residents, the porter, any workman and even the police went to her with any problems, with the expectation, usually fulfilled, that she would solve them. According to Helen Gough, a radiographer and fellow resident, it was a huge responsibility. She was a staunch supporter of the Keyboard Trust a charity for young musicians, she loved the cinema and going to the theatre, and often organised outings for members of staff and students.

Marion's life was truly exceptional, her involvement in the radiographic world, both domestically and internationally, legend. She was a wonderful, loyal and supportive friend. She was full of energy, determined, always focused on the job in hand, ambitious for those under her charge, generous to a fault with time and emotion, mean with herself, unsympathetic to the foolish and lazy. She worked incredibly hard even after her retirement, and she inspired an enormous love and respect.

Postscript

On 1 April, 2004 (April Fool's Day!), aged 83, in typical fashion, Marion set up another working party, this time to gather together a history of the Schools of Radiography and Radiotherapy at The Middlesex Hospital, as, with the closure of the hospital,

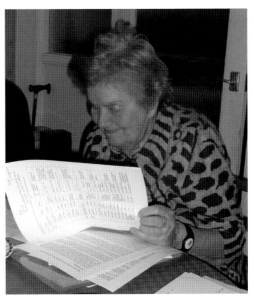

Image 70: Marion studying the working party papers, Heron Court, 2010

she was afraid it would be lost. There was no thought then of a book. Until the last year she hosted all the meetings at her flat, provided food, read all the papers and had enormous input. It was decided to write a book. Sadly, just as it was coming to fruition her death, on 15 September 2011, was announced. Two weeks later, as the editor was bullying all the authors to produce their copy there was a plaintive phone call from a contributor, "She's still pulling our strings". She will be sorely missed.

CHAPTER 6

Memories

The information for this chapter is an amalgam of the wonderful memories, written, emailed, recorded, telephoned and recounted in casual conversations, with much laughter at 'book committee meetings', and to members of the committee on other occasions. They tell of an enormously amusing and enjoyable life, the fun leading to a team spirit which the Schools felt was second to none.

For many, working and studying at The Middlesex was incredibly hard. One secretary probably expressed what many felt, that London and The Middlesex could be a bit of a culture shock whether you came from rural Norfolk, a small village in India, a not-very-well-funded hospital in Nigeria, or even a more relaxed district hospital in England. It took many three months or more to adapt to the language and culture, to a more formal, structured environment and an old, dark, wood-lined department with strong traditions. An ability to read

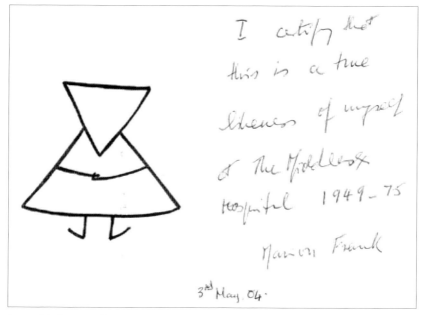

Image 71: Cartoon of Marion Frank certified by Marion as a true representation

Marion Frank's handwriting helped a great deal, and in the early days of one's employment understanding what she said could be a challenge. There was an occasion at a European meeting when even the interpreter asked what language the lady was speaking. The staff had a lot to learn from the many postgraduate students from all over the world studying for the Higher or Teacher's Diploma. They added to the richness of experience and led to some long-standing friendships. Life was not without its humour. One newly-appointed secretary received a phone call purporting to come from a newly-arrived international postgraduate student at Heathrow airport. He had an almost impenetrable accent and said he was due to start at Middlesex that day; he had arrived with his four wives and ten children with a commensurate number of suitcases. Where was his accommodation? Marion had just left for some international meeting and was unavailable. Of course it was all a practical joke by John Twydle, himself newly-appointed to the staff and a past radiography student, but only an exaggeration of what did happen on many occasions.

The many visiting lecturers always had something to add, whether they got trapped in the recalcitrant lift (the engineers, who lived on the ground floor, were used to having to release people), or were like the absent minded ultra-sound lecturer from Leeds, who forgot she had brought her eight year old son with her and left him in the kitchen, whilst she travelled home. There was also one, searching the rabbit warren that was the School for where he was supposed to be lecturing, who wrote an official letter of complaint to Marion when he found a senior member of the teaching staff in the kitchen 'slurping her tea out of her saucer'.

Most past teachers and staff at the School are steadfast in their view that one of the prerequisites of getting employment there was an ability to cater for large numbers of people, though typing came a not so distant second. Indeed Jenny Davidson (Richmond) (1971-1973) reports that her interview consisted of drinking sherry and being asked about how well she could cook and cater for large numbers. She was in, as she had completed a cordon bleu cookery course. Barbara Turner (Allen) (1982-1990) remembers going to Margaret McClellan for careers' advice and being offered a job; in 1964 Adrienne Finch (Bennett) was similarly offered a job when she had phoned up only for the telephone number of a friend with whom she had lost contact. It couldn't be done today; the Human Resources Department would be on the case. Nowadays recruitment and being recruited is not so easy: a great deal more expensive, but of course much more open. Marilyn Swann (Walton) was incredibly grateful to be offered a job as student teacher instantly and on spec which rescued her from a difficult situation at her current workplace. She eventually became Principal of the School of Nuclear Medicine and Ultrasound. She said that the atmosphere in The Middlesex School was unbelievably stimulating ('a frenetic pace of life') and she was determined to justify Marion's faith in her. It enabled her to climb the ladder very fast and Adrienne Finch said the same, becoming a top grade Principal at the age of twenty six.

Marion Frank was excellent at making sure that those whom she wanted on the staff who had family commitments could fit their home life in. Adrienne remembers being allowed to work two days a week from 10-4 and no school holidays, because she could tutor in physics. Her hours gradually increased until she became Deputy to Marion Frank. Then notification was received that for the first time in history, the Schools were to be inspected by the College of Radiographers. The students were told that when they saw the College inspectors in private they could say anything, but not that the Deputy was part-time, which was against College regulations (the TC document again!). One tutor, not having sorted out her child care, had the baby in a cot in her office and the other staff entertained him whilst she did her lectures. One overseas postgraduate student asked permission to name his newly arrived baby sister after a teacher whom he respected. Despite the hard work, trials and tribulations most look back at the years in the Schools as a happy and exciting time. People felt they were at the centre of things.

Between the 1940s and 1960s there were eight students per set, all female, admitted twice a year. Up to 1950 the training was dual (therapy and diagnostic) and on their first day four students were sent to radiotherapy and four to diagnostic. A quick talk from whoever was in charge (sister or superintendent radiographer), and they were attached to a senior student and learnt by following her. Nowadays this would be called, with some scorn, 'the sitting next to Nellie method'.

In Theo Gibbs' set in 1947 there were four ex-service personnel and four school leavers, plus two nurses (Sister Margaret Wells and Sister Marjorie Tomlinson, the latter always known as 'Tommy'). Tommy, a firm Catholic, apparently always gave up sweets for Lent, but saved her ration coupons and had a big binge after

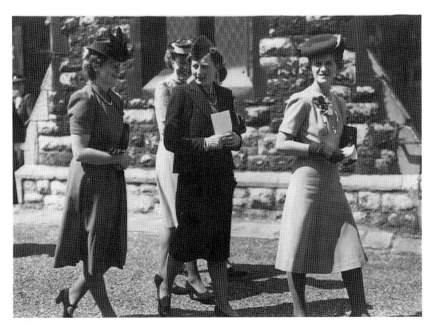
Image 72: 1940s students

Easter! Theo said that in the late 1940s, when despite the war having ended, the country was deeply in debt, and the appalling winter of 1947 led to many power cuts, and, possibly because of the poor condition of the civilian population, a major outbreak of influenza: 'It was a nightmare, the relief of arriving at the hospital each morning where it was warm was overwhelming. Travelling in the cold was a feat of endurance'. She also remembers there being no functioning lifts because of a power failure and the student's role when assigned to 'mobile x-rays' being to run up eight flights of stairs with the lead-lined cassettes for a hip pinning in the operating theatre and down again for them to be processed in the basement. There would have been at least four trips each way. Theo remained slim all her life!

Fees were paid (40 guineas in the first year (£915), 30 guineas (£685) in the second). Home Nursing and First Aid certificates were required and students had to buy their own uniforms from Bourne and Hollingsworth on Oxford Street. These were plain white button-through, cotton, with a white belt (later changed to light blue canvas), little Sister Dora caps, tan lace-up shoes and

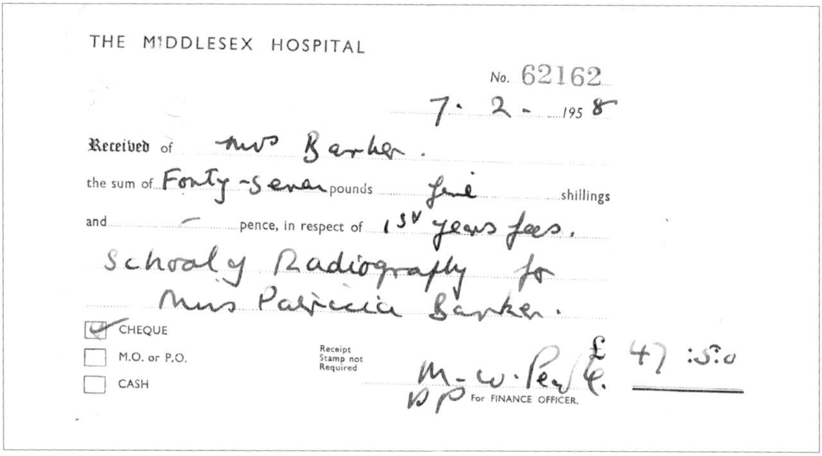

THE MIDDLESEX HOSPITAL

No. 62162

7 - 2 - 195 8

Received of ~nw² *Barker* .

the sum of **Forty - Seven** pounds *five* .... shillings

and .... pence, in respect of 1st *years fees,*

School of Radiography for
Mrs Patricia Barker .

☑ CHEQUE

☐ M.O. or P.O.

☐ CASH

Receipt
Stamp not
Required

M - W. *Peak* £ 47 :5:0

For FINANCE OFFICER.

Image 73: Receipt for fees, 1958

stockings (never to be removed even in the hottest of weather). The first time the students asked to dispense with the caps was in 1951, and the request was summarily turned down; they were not finally disposed of until 1973 despite further requests. The caps were hated: they were stiff and uncomfortable, if you had short hair they would not stay on, and woe betide you if Matron caught you improperly dressed. The uniforms were laundered by the hospital laundry and were so well starched that they could almost stand up on their own and could be very sore and uncomfortable at the neck. For the diagnostic students, the chemical fixer used in film processing (sodium thiosulphate in acid), stained the uniforms badly, and you certainly could not afford to buy new ones. The removable buttons had to be taken out before the dress went to the wash and it was extraordinarily difficult to get them back into the starched cotton. At one stage the staff had double-fronted uniforms and had twenty-two buttons to change. These often got lost and they went rusty if they were left in during washing. The shoes

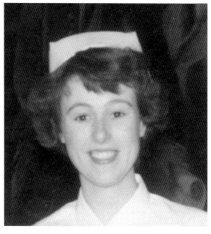

Image 74: A student wearing a Sister Dora cap

151

were quite smart when you first bought them, but films dripping photographic chemicals all and every day rotted the leather, crystallised the shoes, and smelt appalling. If students were working in a very dark fluoroscopy room (where, before the days of image intensifiers the only light was very low level red) they kept their shoes loosely laced so they could slop about, making plenty of noise so people could hear them coming even if they could not see them. Those who tanned easily used to draw a line up the back of their legs to look like stocking seams and often got away with it. Students were not allowed to travel home or go on to Oxford Street in uniform, but it was not unheard of for a complaint to be made by Bourne and Hollingsworth, so there is a great deal of doubt as to whether this edict was always obeyed. Life in the departments was very formal, first names between students or staff were strictly forbidden, the wearing of any jewellery was prohibited.

In 1951 the Nursing Education Committee first mooted the idea of having blazers for the radiography and physiotherapy students. After much discussion on colour, Cambridge blue was chosen for the radiography students and green for physiotherapists. The embroidered hospital badge, with its motto 'miseris succurrere disco' was emblazoned on the left pocket. The actual translation of this motto is 'I learn to help the sick', though many thought it more appropriate as 'miserable suckers with slipped disks'. Graham Gardner, the tailors, came in and measured the students for the blazers, which were useful and worn with much pride. No other school had such an item of uniform, and to a degree they gave students a feeling of esteem. They finally went when the Schools merged with UCH school in 1982, when blazers fell out of fashion and elitism became unpopular. The hierarchical structure of the staffing at The Middlesex, the blazers, and the formality of address made others feel that Middlesex staff and students thought themselves to be a cut above the rest. Thirty years later, on the merger of The Middlesex and University College Schools, there was endless discussion on what uniform would be worn by the students and what colour the belts should be. Finally, it was decided that a delightful deep brown should be used, which resulted in some unfortunate comments relating to bodily waste.

Up to 1967 the students changed in a large basement room under Outpatients in Cleveland Street. This had been a workhouse in both the Georgian and

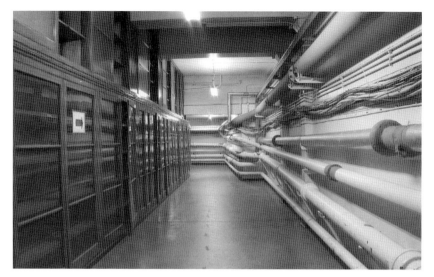
Image 75: Underground tunnels

Victorian eras. The room was desperately overcrowded, with radiography and physiotherapy students and records staff changing there, and was dank, dark and smelly. At the end of a working day, it stank of sweat, fixer and feet. Marion Frank had no sense of smell and did not understand what the complaints were about. There was a long walk to the department, underground through the basement of Outpatients, under Cleveland Street, with turn-offs to the Bland Sutton Institute (biochemistry) and the John Astor nurses' home. The tunnels were very hot, lined with enormous pipes, carrying who knows what, and glass fronted cupboards containing leather bound, ancient ledgers. It was eerie, particularly at night (one never knew who might be round the next corner), but better than braving the cold outdoors in a short sleeved uniform. One secretary was always coming back to the school having delivered the mail to the post room soaking wet. She finally admitted that she was terrified of the basement corridors and of getting lost, never to resurface. Having been shown the route and the markers to be used she found the only problem was avoiding the cockroaches.

Lectures took place at various times during the day, except on Friday afternoons or Saturday mornings, which were free for students on alternate weeks. The students arranged this rota themselves and one set of seven students realised that as long as three were in the department on each half day it was unlikely that anyone would check whether there should be a fourth, so every eight weeks there was a blessed long weekend arranged on a strict rota. In two years they were never found out! Anatomy lectures were initially given by the consultant radiologists, and in the 1940s one student recalls a lecture being illustrated by a male medical student in the 'bare flesh'. Someone complained to Sister Craig and the episode was not repeated!

Preliminary examinations were held at three months and included staff reports to assess suitability, followed by a terrifying interview with Matron. There was no appeal. If you did not pass or were otherwise deemed unsuitable you could not continue. One student who expected a poor report and to be out was praised by the then Matron, Miss Marjorie Marriott (1946-1965) who did not realise that she had confused two students with the same surname. She did not admit her mistake and both students stayed. The Middlesex Schools had the tradition of students taking the Part 1 and Part 2 qualification examinations together. However if you failed one subject in Part 1, you had to retake the whole of Part 2 again as well, even if you had actually passed them all; it was the only training school to do this. Fortunately, the College of Radiographers' edict later banned this iniquitous practice. The prize giving for successful students was held for many years jointly with the physiotherapy students and many famous people presented these prizes. Lewis Douglas, the US Ambassador, did so in 1949, Princess Margaret in 1950, Viscount Montgomery of Alamein in 1951, the Duke of Northumberland (1952 & 1960), Sir Edmund Hillary in 1953 - the year he climbed Mount Everest with Sherpa Tenzing Norgay, the Queen Mother (1955), Princess Alexandra (1958) and Sir Malcolm Sargent (1959).

As a new student, whether in diagnostic or radiotherapy, one's first job was cleaning, making sure all the equipment and control panels were clean and tidy. The cleaners did not like washing the floor under the examination tables as they thought the x-rays were produced continuously and this area was dangerous so when that area got really dirty, the students cleaned that too. In the diagnostic department one spent a lot of time carrying heavy, lead lined cassettes to and from the darkroom as the overhead carrier (state of the art in 1935) was, by 1957, always getting stuck, and no one would use it for fear of a patient's films being abandoned there for hours until a step ladder and a strong man could be found to rescue them. The other task was trailing around after the radiology registrars trying to get them to check out the wet films once produced. Having trainee radiologists meant that radiographers could not check out their own films to ensure they were of diagnostic quality before being able to send patients home, which appeared to be the norm everywhere else. It could all take hours, and if a patient needed a repeat film, it was nothing for them to stay half a day for a simple chest x-ray. The introduction of automatic processing was a life-changing event in diagnostic radiography, as patients often left the department in half an hour, instead of a minimum of two hours. The staff in the Casualty Department complained that the

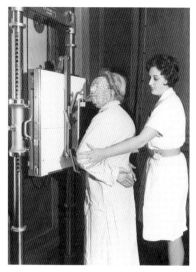

Image 76: Performing a chest x-ray

patients were coming back too quickly as they had got used to blaming the X-ray Department for patient delays and often emptied their own waiting rooms by sending patients for x-ray, whether necessary or not. There were no targets for waiting times then!

In the late 1950s it was quite usual to do a chest x-ray on over one hundred patients a day. Many were from the heart and cancer wards and very ill, but all outpatients coming in for surgery and all maternity patients had a routine chest x-ray. Two weeks, twice a year were given over to doing a chest x-ray (on the mass miniature machine) on every single member of staff and medical student (about 5000). This was before the days of Alice Stewart's seminal paper on the possibility of the induction of childhood leukaemia caused by in utero exposure, before knowledge of the risks associated with low-dose radiation was widespread and before a cost benefit analysis had to be performed before any request for x-ray examination was made. It was a department rule that every patient had to be accompanied from the waiting room on the ground floor to the chest examination room in the basement. One student, Anne Mackereth (Winterton), wore a pedometer for a week and found she had averaged twelve miles each day. After all this students were supposed to go home and study. Many just fell asleep, particularly if they had had an hour's journey on a crowded tube.

155

It was incredibly busy, but the technicalities could be undemanding with so many routine chest x-rays to be done on fit patients. Repeating the same instruction, forty or fifty times a day, five days a week only remains interesting if one can focus on achieving the ultimate, 'every patient should feel that they are the first of the day'. Students learnt to say 'breathe in and hold it' in a variety of languages, and sometimes forgot to say 'breathe out' until the patient was close to exploding. So many patients do exactly what they are told: 'Go in this cubicle, undress completely and put this gown on over your head', only for the student to find that they have given the patient a pillow case instead of a gown and the patient has done exactly what they were told. Male patients regularly queried how they were going to take their trousers off if they could keep their shoes and socks on. It was also very important to check the patient's name carefully to make quite sure you had the correct person. The patients would be nervous and respond to any name, anxious not miss their turn. There was the memorable occasion when a private patient attending for a lumbar spine x-ray did just this and ended up having a barium enema, and all the staff laughed politely when he said the examination was nothing like he expected. To cap it all the films were chewed up by the processor. The patient who should have had the barium enema was found quietly sitting in the waiting room. At the end of the day one had to ensure that all the cubicles had been checked, for sometimes an obedient patient would still be there, waiting to be sent away, for the radiographer-on-call to find at some ungodly hour of the night.

The Middlesex, along with other London teaching hospitals, was often at the forefront of developing new treatments for diseases or investigating new diseases. One of the contributors to this book says the following: 'One of my saddest memories of being a student, which is still carried with me today, was dealing with a young man with HIV at the end of his life. It was the early 1980s, HIV was just being recognised and little was known about it. So little that we all had to gown and glove up and go to the patients in isolation. The patient was confused because of the stage of the disease, and bitterly lonely and distressed because of the isolation and lack of physical contact. He hadn't been able to tell his family because of the stigma, and he didn't get comfort from the staff because everyone was so frightened'.

Some radiography students, and of course staff, acquired strain and other injuries which to an extent stayed with them all their lives. There was one tale of the acquisition of a lifelong neck injury. In those days there were not the same rules about lifting patients then as there are now and this was a classic case of the radiographer keen to get home, of the last patient of the day, a small, elderly lady needing to get back to the ward in a wheel chair, and all the porters being busy. One careless lift, feeling the pop as two discs in the neck slipped out of position, excruciating pain, six weeks off work and being sent £14 compensation by a government department. It was a problem that lasted the whole of this student's working life. Apart from repetitive strain injury, the other problem in the early days was dermatitis from the wet chemicals, and even when automatic processing became the norm, asthma caused by the inhalation of chemicals in the atmosphere. These latter two conditions sometimes meant that you could not continue your training or profession. Nowadays things are so much better.

According to Ann Paris (1964-1969), life whether as staff or student, was never dull. Although the 'esprit de corps' of the Schools was firmly founded on the quality of the education for both staff and students, enjoying oneself was an important part of working at The Middlesex. As early as 1948, Theo Gibbs recalls that London, post-war and despite rationing, enabled a social life with staff dances in York House on Berners Street and a good selection of cinemas and theatres to choose from. She recalls that restaurants were restricted to charging no more than five shillings (£5.70p) for a meal. In the 1960s a student remembers Matron being the provider of free tickets for West End shows, which were available after 4.30pm once the nurses had had first pick. Many students and radiographers have fond memories of evenings spent at the theatre in posh seats for free and one remembers an unforgettable visit on complimentary tickets to the front stalls at Covent Garden to see Margot Fonteyn and Rudolf Nureyev dance in *The Nutcracker*. However, in the era before grants, many students lived at home to spare the expense of living in Marlborough Court and this, they felt, did curtail their social life. This included missing out on enjoying 'a half pint of bitter and a roast beef sandwich' at the Swan around the corner from the residence at Marlborough Court, all for two shillings and sixpence (£1.60), remembers Mary Pluister.

In the late fifties student radiographers were not allowed to join the student societies associated with the medical school. However the Christian Union, the Choir and for some reason the Fencing Club were open to them. One student was Captain of the Fencing Club team for a short time, and talented and good looking students could even get into the cast for the Medical School Christmas Cabaret. However one student, Adrienne Finch, managed to become an honorary member of the medical school, she thinks by turning up at an annual hospital sports day with a pair of running spikes, so the powers-that-be thought she must know what she was doing. The Middlesex Hospital Medical School was short of female competitors so she was invited to participate in the London Inter-Hospital Sports Day and attend training at the Highgate Harriers ground. She was entered for six events including the shot putt and discus, neither of which she had ever done before. Her athletics career was curtailed when she realised that her right biceps was a great deal larger than the left and she couldn't take seriously a female competitor who cried when she couldn't achieve her target time for the hundred yard sprint. Life working in the hospital could be tough enough without making more hurdles for oneself.

Again at a similar time, there were annual swimming and tennis matches between the physiotherapy and radiography students, for which cups were presented. The radiography students always had difficulty raising a team for either and were usually beaten. Compared with the physiotherapists, apart from the odd enthusiast, they were not a sporty lot and thought that physiotherapists took life far too seriously.

Some of the enjoyment took place jointly with other schools of radiography. For many years there was an annual London and Home Counties' students' sports day, with every school of radiography sending in a team and where none of the races was regarded seriously, with fancy dress, buckets of water, silly games and laughter being de rigueur. There were races involving stretchers and all sorts of other medical equipment; and certainly an amount of alcohol was consumed. One notable year the teachers' rounders team was disqualified for cheating (they had three extra team members!). The only school that treated the event seriously was the Army school, with its unbelievably fit and disciplined students, until they realised that the organiser for the following year was the school which had won on the previous occasion. At this point they joined the anarchy of the others and worked at losing.

One set of radiotherapy students decided to enter as a team in the *Sunday Times* fun run. The whole set participated, calling themselves "The Radioactive Saucies".

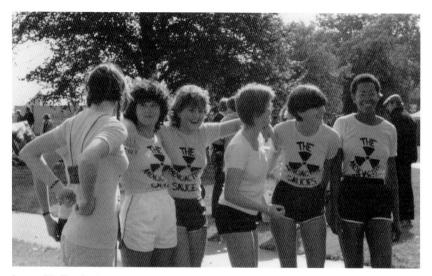

Image 77: The Radioactive Saucies

Team T-shirts were stencilled, with the radiation symbol and the team name. They had so much fun that they decided to enter the next year and jokingly suggested that as it was a School of Radiotherapy Team, Mary Embleton, as Principal should be part of the team. She decided to accept their challenge and even managed to complete the run in a shorter time than at least one of the students!

The opening of the Schools' new premises in Foley Street in 1967 was celebrated with a great party and it goes without saying this was masterminded by Marion Frank. At the time Marion was President of the Society/College and never one to miss a fund raising opportunity; any party profit was to go towards the Society's furniture fund for their new premises. Each floor of the Schools had a different theme; the first floor was a Strawberry Garden serving strawberries and cream, which Marion had been up at the crack of dawn visiting Convent Garden to buy. The second floor was a pub selling beer and frankfurters and there were skittles and darts to be played. On the top floor there was a disco: on the door was a Dutch nun who was a trained radiographer working in the X-ray Department at the time, and who ensured that no one got in without paying. The whole event was a huge success, attended not only by the department staff, but many from the rest of the hospital as well as personnel from The Society of Radiographers.

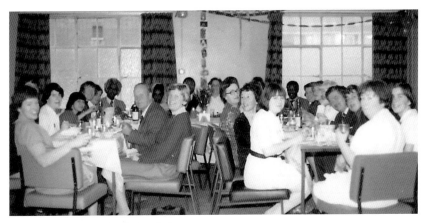

Image 78: Christmas lunch, fourth floor

Food for many of the parties was usually procured from Schmidt's in Charlotte Street because of their splendid range of German sausages. The frankfurters would be steamed in a specially adapted steriliser which prevented them from boiling, 'borrowed' from the department. Its previous purpose had been to sterilise the metal enema catheters! One Christmas the party on the fourth floor went particularly well with the alcohol flowing freely. Marion Frank had arranged for the partygoers to attend the Medical School Christmas Show and as she announced it was time to go over to take up the seats she began to distribute bars of chocolate to the inebriated. Sue Boult, a School Secretary, says she has never forgotten Marion's advice that chocolate counteracts the effects of alcohol!

The Christmas lunch each year was a major event. Marion Frank was the inspiration and staff were allocated the many tasks. This lunch was used as a way to thank all those who had helped the school during the year and there was much competition to receive an invitation. Many outside lecturers came, as did all the international post-diploma students, for many of whom it was their first introduction to a Christmas dinner. For those who missed home at this time it was a great and very happy celebration; there could be as many as one hundred guests. Turkey, ham, stuffing, roast potatoes, brussel sprouts, gravy, cranberry sauce, Christmas pudding (steamed in the steriliser of course), mince pies, everything was produced out of the small kitchen on the fourth floor. Dinners were also held at the end of a weekend course, and one staff member remembers producing profiteroles, cream and chocolate sauce with a choice of apple cake

160

for eighty. How no guests were given food poisoning is a mystery but the meals were great fun and a superb opportunity to build the team spirit.

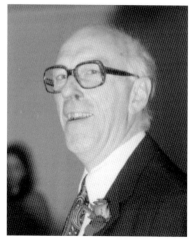

Lindy's cake shop in Mortimer Street is remembered by many students and staff members. Dr Graham Whiteside would press a small sum into the palm of a student to go and buy cream cakes for the tea break during an afternoon urodynamics session, and others recall Saturday mornings ending in a trip over the road for sticky buns. There was a twenty-first birthday celebration for the radiographer in Accident

Image 79: Dr Graham Whiteside

and Emergency, champagne and chocolate cake during a quiet moment in the working day. This would be a reason for dismissal now but was a happy occasion, fondly remembered. There was also the Glory café 'across the road', run by Greek Cypriots, whose territory Cleveland Street then was, and who provided omelette and chips with everything for two and six (£1.90p).

Most of the entertainment took place in the school but one student, Ann Mackereth, recalls an eventful student trip to the Brussels Exhibition in 1958:

We were to fly from Blackbushe Airfield in Hampshire quite early in the morning but had to wait for ages before taking off, which was a bit disturbing, but eventually arrived in Brussels rather later than we had expected. Four of us went up to the top of the Atomium on the escalators, but then were still there when they closed and we had to go down the most frightening external fire escape. At which point Marion Frank was overcome with an acute attack of vertigo. The story goes that this was soon remedied by a medicinal dose of brandy but the adventure wasn't over. The return flight was plagued by turbulence and the landing back at Blackbushe was in the dark. The passengers were then kept for some time from disembarking without anyone understanding what was happening until eventually the door was opened and a handful of pyjama-clad men appeared asking why

161

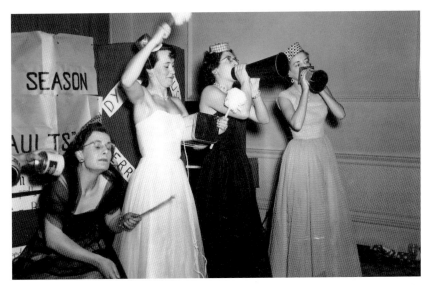

Image 80: Marlborough Court cabaret in the 1950s, June Penney (Legg) second from left

the plane had landed at RAF Odiham, ten miles from Blackbushe! The flight then took off again and landed at the correct airfield, with Marion Frank as charterer responsible for all the landing fees. It is believed that Brigadier Hardy Roberts, the Hospital's Secretary Superintendent, got her out of that one! (He later became Comptroller of the Queen's Household).

From 1960 onwards there was a Christmas dance held at Marlborough Court. As part of the tradition which continued right up to the closure of the school, some sort of a cabaret was produced at most School and Department celebrations by the staff and students. Once the top floor of the new premises were available, parties and social occasions became more than an annual event. These included one to mark the retirement of Dr Graham Whiteside. It included a song adapted by Richard Evans: 'I right the wrongs that make the whole world sick, for urine problems I'm the man to pick' was performed to a big Barry Manilow hit 'I write the songs that make the whole world sing...'.

Richard also produced a version of the song Maggie May, which was dedicated to Margaret McClellan (the Deputy Principal at the time). 'Oh Maggie I think I've got something to say to you....'. Richard became famous for his impersonation of Marion Frank at her retirement party, complete with oversized three cornered hat

162

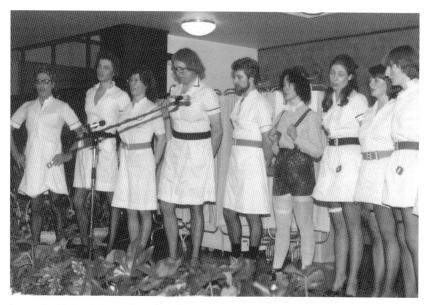

Image 81: Cabaret chorus line of students, staff, radiologists and physicists

and distinctive walk. He was bribed to travel to the Teachers' seminar that year to repeat the performance, which brought the house down. He had to be promised that it would not affect his employment prospects as many of his likely future employers were present; he later went on to become chief executive of the Society and College of Radiographers.

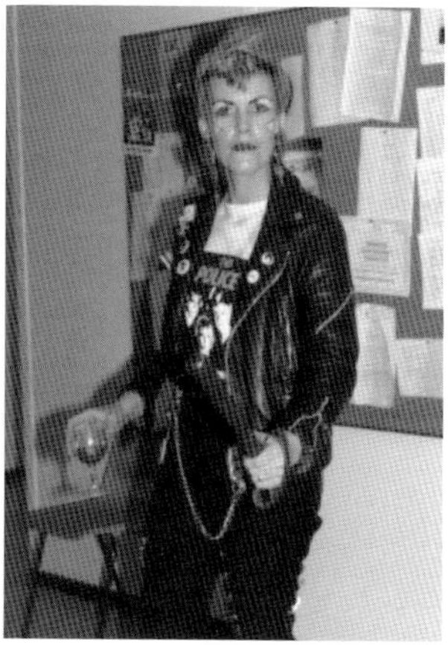

Fancy dress parties were popular in the 1980s. The Imaging Department Superintendent Jean Harvey dressed up as the most convincing punk rocker at one of these, and Tom Bryant, a physicist, was part of a chorus line which went on stage, the men in drag, in very short skirts, suspenders and black fishnet stockings .

Opportunities for practical jokes were taken whenever they arose. Adrienne Finch recalls the pride taken by Brigadier Geoffrey Hardy-Roberts, the Secretary Superintendent (nowadays he

Image 82: Jean Harvey ready to party as a punk rocker

163

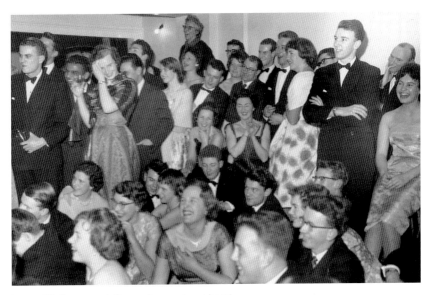
Image 83: An appreciative audience at a cabaret

would be called the Chief Executive), in the courtyard lawn and the Monday morning inspections he undertook with Matron, complete with starched lace, frilly cap and flying cape. The radiography department were nefariously involved in a plot by the medical students who sowed this lawn with mustard and cress and then led him to believe that as the lawn was adjacent to the x-ray department, the x-rays were obviously causing his grass to mutate.

Students also recall taking part in events of national significance. Marjorie Moyle remembers in 1944 students being given 'Victory in Europe' (VE day) off to join the crowds celebrating in central London at the end of the Second World War. In 1960 when Princess Margaret married Anthony Armstrong-Jones, Middlesex students waved their scarves at the best man, Roger Gilliatt, a neurological consultant at the Hospital and nearly two decades later, in 1981, the students celebrated the wedding of HRH the Prince of Wales to Lady Diana Spencer. One student recalls that the organisation was fairly spontaneous and began with a plan to attend the fireworks in Hyde Park on the eve of the wedding. Stephanie Williamson (Farley) recalls:

We got so caught up in the excitement that after leaving the park (by climbing over the railings to avoid the queues) we rushed back to the

Nurses' Home in Gower St, grabbed blankets and headed for the Mall. We pitched ourselves on the pavement and spent the night singing patriotic songs (although I do remember trying to sleep but the pavement was too hard) and found ourselves in a marvellous position to watch the event unfold. The best bit was abandoning the blankets and rushing down the Mall for the famous balcony scene and being surprised how little we could see because the balcony really is a long way off! I am not sure how we accounted for the missing blankets but I am sure we must have done because in those days the laundry was strictly administered and accounted for. We would get one clean sheet a week and you had to rotate the used sheet down to the mattress and use the clean one for the upper sheet!

The Middlesex Hospital attracted patients from all walks of life, from the Greek Cypriot seamstresses who worked in the local dress factories to members of the landed gentry. One patient who had quite an impact on the hospital and the X-ray Department in particular was Sir Winston Churchill. In May 1962 he was at his home in Monaco when he fell and fractured the neck of his femur, and it was decided he should be brought to The Middlesex Hospital to have the femur pinned. Once the news was announced the whole hospital seemed to be in a dither: everything had to be in place for his arrival, a private room in the Woolavington Wing was cleared and cleaned, the operating theatre was prepared, the x-ray machines were in place before he had left Monaco. The press filled the front entrance hall, with the brass-buttoned, tail-coated ex-servicemen who were porters trying to keep them under control. The journalists were finally given an office off the front hall although students and staff remember finding journalists forever lurking in corridors and corners, trying to get a member of staff to give them a quote. Of course x-rays of the fracture would be required on admission, in the operating theatre and on several occasions subsequently. Sir Winston's short, rotund stature was not one to make any x-ray easy and to ensure everything went without a hitch some trial exposures took place. A well-built security guard stood outside the theatre, he was of similar build to Sir Winston, so he was drafted in and x-ray films were taken of him fully dressed and the gun in his pocket was duly revealed. Sir Winston was renowned for his colourful language and Dr Frederick Campbell Golding, the Director of the department, banned 'the girls' from x-raying the great man because of this, so Marion Frank was directed to take on the role of the lowly radiographer on mobiles. Even she could not get him to hold his breath. Lady Churchill would visit him every evening, passing down the X-ray Department corridor, and despite her concern, she never failed to acknowledge the on-call radiographer. Sir Winston was discharged from hospital on Wednesday 22 August 1962, and once again there was a great commotion, with crowds filling Cleveland Street. Marion had banned anyone from watching or recording the occasion, but she was found out when the *Daily Telegraph* published a picture of her

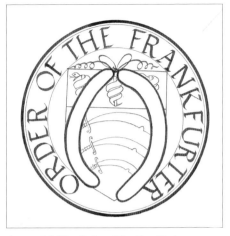

Image 84: The Order of the Frankfurter

leaning dangerously out of a window, using a cine camera to image the event.

In 1980 the school celebrated Marion Frank's award of the OBE. The event was marked by another 'frankfurters-in-the-steriliser party' and the issuing of the 'Order of the Frankfurter' to every participant. Apart from an ability to cook for five thousand, Marion Frank was a superb judge of character; she could always see what people could do if pushed, and she pushed them. She found out what other skills staff and students might have and the founding of the hospital radio in 1981 by a student radiographer was just such an occasion.

As a new student, Stephanie Farley had been disappointed that a radio station did not already exist and Marion Frank challenged her to change that state of affairs. She was even offered Wednesday afternoons (officially the time for training for those involved in the hospital sports teams) to work on the project. It was quite a daunting prospect. However the temptation was too great and she soon found herself in the office of Alan Langlands who was Unit Administrator at the time. He set a handful of targets: show that patients wanted a radio station; find a place for it and garner support for funding. Thankfully Marion, who was Chair of the Middlesex Hospital League of Friends, looked after the last, and a large room in the basement under the hospital shop was identified as a suitable location. A minor league professional radio presenter was persuaded to pre-record a show for broadcast and with

166

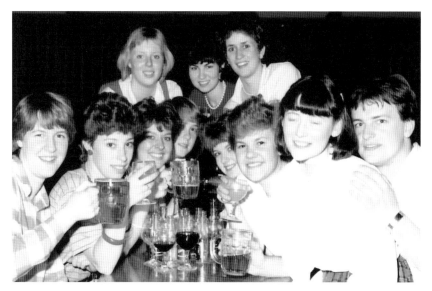

Image 85: Middlesex students enjoying their first conference in the early 1980s

some very basic equipment, the volunteers, who were supplemented by technical expertise from the BBC in Portland Place, were able to intercept the bedside radio system and play the show to the patients whilst they were surveyed! Thankfully the one hour show was incredibly good and patients liked it. The League of Friends equipped the studio, and a high profile official opening was held in 1981 in the hospital boardroom, with special guests Joe Bugner (the champion heavyweight boxer), Bonnie Langford (the actress and dancer) and Gertrude Schilling (famous for her hats). The radio station was soon broadcasting seven days a week and went on to complete stunts such as a week-long non-stop broadcast from the front car park of the hospital and interviews with celebrities including the cast of *Cats*, which was London's biggest show at the time. Another radiography student, Richard Evans, adapted Dickens' *A Christmas Carol* for the radio and the team went on to record it using celebrities, hospital consultants, staff and patients as cast members.

Interaction with the medical school did improve, and by the 1970s radiography students were participating in Freshers' Week including the 'Hit Squad' who could be hired for a small fee to throw shaving foam pies at individuals. The hit list was published in advance so that the target had the opportunity to 'reverse' the hit for a further sum. Students began to put together teams to enter the famous Freshers' Week Treasure Hunt. This generally involved careering around central London stealing famous street signs (the better known the greater the points) and kidnapping unsuspecting passers by (the more daring, the more points) and bringing them back to the student union bar. Stephanie Farley remembers scoring quite a few points for the roll that has the names of all the stops from the front end of a double decker bus. She can't quite recall how she came to acquire it but knows it headed off to Australia in a radiographer's shipping crate!

The authors wonder in these days of frantically busy and 'cost effective' departments whether students and staff ever have time to relax and to take part in activities which help bonding and build team spirit. There is separation of the delivery of the theoretical components of the course at a university with very large intakes from the clinical sites, where the student groups are often far apart from each other in distant hospitals. There seems to be no 'time out', no opportunity for plots to be hatched, 'in jokes' told and activities planned. Will the modern student fondly remember their training days as past radiographers do?

CHAPTER 7

The Merger and the End

The 1980s was a decade of change in radiography education, both nationally and at The Middlesex Hospital. At the beginning of 1980 Professor Roger Berry was elected Chairman of the Radiography Education Committee and the membership and accountability of the committee was reviewed and agreed in consultation with the District Administrator, Mr Tony Knowles; Julia Lovell was promoted to the position of Principal (at grade 2) in charge of the School of Nuclear Medicine and Medical Ultrasound. The impending retirement of Marion Frank was a catalyst for the inspection of the Schools by the College of Radiographers in February 1980. As the body responsible for awarding professional qualifications, the College of Radiographers set standards for schools of radiography and regularly inspected them to check that they complied. The Middlesex Hospital's Schools had not previously been inspected, probably due to Marion Frank and Mary Craig's having been very actively involved in the work of the College. Documentation prepared for the visit is held in the University College London Hospitals' archives, and includes lists of the Schools' accommodation and equipment at the time. Marion wanted everything to be perfect before she left.

The inspection report made no adverse comments but gave a number of recommendations. The Diagnostic School was approved for twenty-four students per annum, whilst the Radiotherapy School, which a couple of years previously had decided to discontinue the March intake and just have one intake of students each year, had its approved intake of students reduced by two, to ten students, until such time as further clinical experience could be provided. Since the closure of Marlborough Court there had been problems finding sufficient living accommodation for students and the recommendation 'that residential accommodation should be provided for all students who require it for the whole period of training', strengthened the Schools' pleas to the district health authority when, in 1984, only twenty-seven beds were being provided, though sixty-five were required. Provision of sufficient accommodation remained a problem right up to the closure of the Schools.

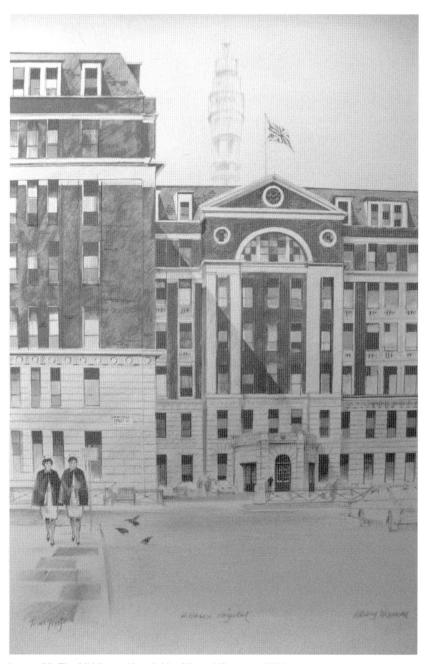

Image 86: The Middlesex Hospital by Albany Wiseman, 1981

While it had been known for some time that Marion Frank would be retiring at the end of 1980, Anne Wells, Radiotherapy Principal, announced at the May Education Committee meeting that she would also be leaving, as she was getting married and moving away. This, together with recommendations that the Schools should consider the possibility of appointing one of the Principals to be co-ordinator for all the Schools and that the Diagnostic School should appoint a Clinical Instructor with the role of co-ordinating placements across all departments associated with the School, led to the Schools being renamed The Middlesex Hospital Schools of Radiography (Diagnosis and Therapy), and a new staffing structure being adopted. Since the late 1970s there had been concerns about the large number of small radiography schools and their doubtful viability, especially in radiotherapy, and the possibility of forging closer links with the Hammersmith Hospital, initially for both disciplines and then more specifically for radiotherapy, was explored.

Because of the strong possibility of the Radiotherapy Schools at The Middlesex and Hammersmith merging, the external assessor on the interview panel for the appointment of a new Radiotherapy Principal was Marjorie Moyle, Superintendent of the Radiotherapy Department at the Hammersmith who had been a student at The Middlesex in 1946. The interviews were held on the day Peter Sellers died in the hospital, and someone had to stand in for the Hospital Administrator,

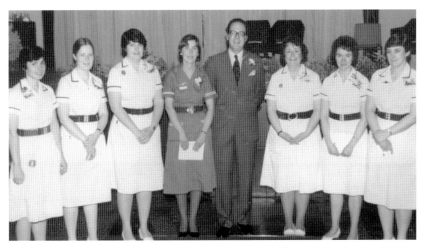

Image 87: The 1985 prize giving: Mary Robinson, Jennifer Edie, Julia Lovell, Mary Embleton, Professor Roger Berry, Margaret McClellan, Mary Lovegrove, Barbara Turner

David Johnson, because he was dealing with the press. Mary Embleton was appointed to the post of Radiotherapy Principal from September 1980.

The selection interviews for the post of Co-ordinating Principal and Head of the Diagnostic section involved all the radiologists, as none would give up his place! Thus the candidates faced eight men and one woman including four radiologists, the Professor of Radiotherapy, a male outside assessor, Donald Graham from Aberdeen, a man from personnel, and Jean Harvey, the Superintendent Radiographer. Margaret McClellan, who was then the Principal at

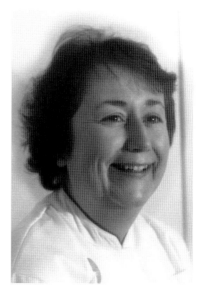

Image 88: Margaret McClellan

St. Bartholomew's Hospital and a previous deputy principal at The Middlesex, took up the position in February 1981.

After Marion Frank retired in December 1980 there was a considerable period of adjustment, not just for the remaining staff and the new Principal, but also for the extended family of lecturers, which included physicists, radiologists and clinical radiographers. Recruitment was becoming difficult, especially for the March intake, and a three year training programme was now compulsory, so the decision was taken in 1982 to withdraw the two-year two-intake programme, and September 1982 saw the first intake to the new three-year, single-intake programme. That, coupled with the upcoming merger with the School at University College Hospital, made for further change.

During 1979, in her final year as Principal, Marion Frank had worked hard at recruiting overseas students and in 1980 there were about seventeen on the books, which was something of a record. They followed courses ranging from three months in administration, to twelve months Further Education Teaching Certificates with clinical updating, or three years of HDCR and TDCR programmes. This meant that all these post-diploma students needed to be in a clinical department which was already fully staffed and supporting a full complement of pre-qualification students. The presence of post-diploma students as well made the patient examination rooms very crowded and occasionally there was competition for the clinical experience. Several of these overseas students needed many hours of teaching practice, and this required much organisation and patience. There was sufficient income generated from them to employ a part-time Clinical Instructor to look after them, and for the first year of her so-called retirement Marion took on that role, and juggled all their needs with those of the Schools and the Department.

The Middlesex Hospital and University College Hospital were less than half a mile apart, with the main thoroughfare of Tottenham Court Road running between them. Both were London Teaching Hospitals with the specialities that such centres of excellence attracted. University College Hospital was founded in 1834, eight years after University College, London (UCL, then known as the London University), in order to provide clinical training for the 'medical classes' of the university, after a refusal by the governors of The Middlesex Hospital to allow students access to their wards. UCL had had what was seen as the presumption to publish as fact that the students studying medicine would be allowed access to The Middlesex Hospital wards without first asking The Middlesex's Board of Governors' permission. The two rival hospitals had thus existed side by side for more than one hundred and fifty years and in the late 1970s it was becoming obvious that some sort of rationalisation was likely, as the money needed to fund two such significant establishments so close to each other would not be continued or afforded forever.

North West Thames Regional Health Authority (NWTRHA) administered The Middlesex Hospital and North East Thames Regional Health Authority (NETRHA) University College Hospital (UCH). Whilst that arrangement continued the threat of rationalisation was remote. In 1982, in one of the many NHS re-organisations, The Middlesex found itself in NETRHA. It was at this point that Alan Langlands became the Unit Administrator of these two major hospitals and was tasked with combining the two centres of excellence at all levels. The Schools of Radiography were one of the first departments to merge, a move precipitated by the impending retirement of Pat Hynes, the Principal at UCH in 1984; the situation was both difficult and delicate. The School at UCH was small compared to that at the Middlesex but some excellent work was being undertaken there. There was no doubt that all the staff, be they radiographic, physics or medical, expected it to be a complete takeover by The Middlesex and it became clear that the clinical staff at UCH were looking for some benefit for themselves in the way of education programmes. Not surprisingly, the Principal at UCH was determined to make her presence felt at all planning meetings and to put the case for UCH at every opportunity. She either did not believe or did not understand that the Middlesex Principal was keen that this should be a merger and not a take-over, and this made for some interesting, if not acrimonious meetings. On one occasion, Barbara Turner, a teacher in the school at The Middlesex, says that she dreaded it when Pat Hynes and Margaret McClellan were in the same room at the same time.

The physicists at The Middlesex were heard to say on more than one occasion that "Marion Frank would not have done or agreed to that". Dr David Edwards, the Chair of the UCH Education Committee, walked out of one meeting stating it was "nothing but a takeover!" Basically it was a no-win situation all round. However, like most storms, when the event became a reality it actually worked well, with little antagonism from either side and a great deal of goodwill from the clinical staff of UCH.

UCH brought to the party a Principal II (a lower grade than the Principal I at The Middlesex), a full-time clinical instructor, an annual intake of eight diagnostic students, a very supportive ultrasound radiologist, and very good physics lecturer. This boosted the complement of staff at The Middlesex and we were able to upgrade the deputy post to a Principal II with special responsibility for overseeing the needs of the department at UCH, and to upgrade the Principal I post to a Principal I with more than twenty-four students. Grading of posts in the health service at that time depended on the size of the student intake.

As University College Hospital had a smaller Radiotherapy Department, which had not been involved in training students, it was immediately clear that the two Departments would amalgamate. One area where the department at UCH had more expertise was in the treatment of children, because of links with Great Ormond Street Hospital for Children, which had no radiotherapy department of its own. Though some staff at UCH were wary of working with students, as they had chosen to work in a non-teaching department, those in charge were keen to forge links with the School and in June 1983 students started going to UCH for clinical experience. Maureen (Mo) Clark, the Superintendent Radiographer, requested a one-year secondment to the Radiotherapy School in order to gain both the Higher and Teacher's Diplomas of the College of Radiographers as part of her professional development. She was seconded as a Student Teacher when the position became vacant in October 1983.

Throughout the 1980s the merger of various departments of the two hospitals continued and the upper echelons of the administration came and went. The Schools of Radiography settled down quite quickly and continued to flourish. March 1984 saw the final group of The Middlesex diagnostic two-year double-intake programme qualify, with one student, Louise Wood, being the thousandth student to go through training since the Schools opened in 1935. The Diploma students now followed the three-year programme with all diagnostic and therapy students at both hospitals following the same Part I programme (Physics, Anatomy, Physiology and Pathology and Care of the Patient - see Appendix A) with the specialist teaching being split between the suitable experts from both hospitals. As before, Part II subjects (for Diagnostic students: Radiographic Equipment, Radiographic Photography and Technique, and for Radiotherapy students: Radiotherapy Physics, Principles of Radiotherapy and Oncology and Radiotherapy Technique) were taught separately (See Appendix A). Staffing levels conformed to the College of Radiographers' requirements and prize-givings were held on the UCH and The Middlesex sites in alternate years.

A new name, uniform and badge were needed to make the merger complete. The title became The Middlesex and UCH Schools of Radiography – sometimes referred to as the Too Much School or even The Much Sex School. The Middlesex blue blazers had become unfashionable, had already been losing favour and were forgotten. There were white uniforms, with coloured belts for the girls and epaulettes for the men. After discussion with the uniform department it was found that the only colour not in use was a delicate shade of brown, perhaps not the ideal choice but it had to do. The Schools' qualification badge was designed and made by Thomas Fattorini.

To begin with the Director of the x-ray department at UCH expressed a wish to continue to be involved with selection of diagnostic students who were to work in his department, but this of course, involved all applicants as they were to gain clinical experience in both departments, and was also a big commitment for someone in his position. Eventually he was unable to give the time and did not take up his place on the newly-formed Education Committee'.

In November 1981, after Marion Frank's retirement, one of the first prize-giving events of the new school was memorable. It was usual to invite a guest to speak to the assembled students, their guests, families and hospital notables. Someone would be chosen who might have a special interest in the Schools, such as a previous student who had become a President of the Society of Radiographers; on one occasion Marion Frank presented prizes to her final intake of students. However, we were keen to break with tradition and invited Dr Rob Buckman, a qualified and practising doctor but also a famous comedian, who broadcast in the popular Pink Medicine show. The current Principal, Margaret McClellan, met him in the Schools and immediately had serious misgivings. As he took off his crash helmet he revealed himself to be a very pleasant young man who clearly did not possess a suit. A collar and tie coupled with a corduroy jacket and jeans was the best he could do! He had been suggested by Professor Roger Berry for this prestigious occasion and Margaret took him to the Courtauld Lecture Theatre where the event was to take place. The platform party, consisting of Margaret McClellan, Mary Embleton, Principal of the Radiotherapy School, Julia Lovell, Principal of the Schools of Medical Ultrasound and Nuclear Medicine, Professor Roger Berry, Chairman of the Education Committee and our guest speaker, ascended the platform to respectful silence from the audience which included Dr John Dunwoody, the Chairman of the Area Health Authority and a past Labour Minister of Health. The normal format continued with reports from the three Principals all introduced by the Chair.

The parents listened eagerly to hear that their offspring had done this, that or the other. The students looked clean, remarkably groomed, unusually tidy and a bit nervous at the thought of having to ascend the stage to collect their certificates. Then it was the turn of the guest speaker. There was keen anticipation in the hall to hear the pearls of wisdom that would surely drop from this member of the medical profession, even if he did not quite look the part. What followed was the most brilliant piece of stand-up comedy, all carefully related to radiography and learning. It is no exaggeration to say that the audience and platform party were crying with laughter. All except, that is, the Chairman of the Area Health

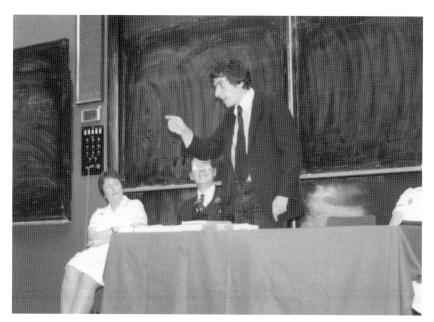

Image 89: Prize giving 1981 with Dr Rob Buckman as guest speaker

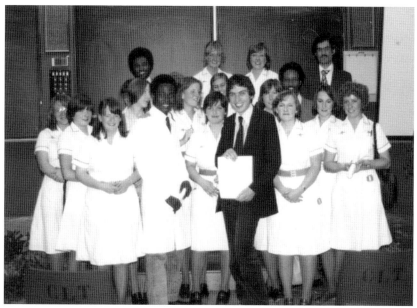

Image 90: The 1981 prize giving: the qualifying students with Dr Rob Buckman

Authority, who sat at the back, stony-faced throughout this brilliant and unusual presentation. The following year's prize-giving was more conventional, with the prizes being presented by Christine Soutter, President of the Society and College of Radiographers and a past student and member of staff.

It was around this time that the name of the Schools changed, in order to recognise all the programmes that were available. The final result was a long-winded title that just about pleased all the relevant parties – The Middlesex and University College Hospitals Schools of Radiography, Radiotherapy and Nuclear Medicine – too much it now definitely was.

The portfolio of courses was complete when in 1984 the Schools started a Higher Diploma Course for radiotherapy radiographers. During the 1970s and early 1980s, Anne Wells and then Mary Embleton had been involved in the pan-London course run by Acton Technical College, but it was no longer in existence. The radiotherapy staffing included a teacher post, which until this time had been filled by a student teacher, but when Mo Clark's secondment ended the School managed to recruit a newly qualified teacher, Judy Taylor, to the post, enabling the Schools to take on the additional commitment of running this post-diploma programme.

1985 saw the fiftieth anniversary of the Schools. A special celebration was planned together with a reunion of previous students. Margaret McClellan and Mary Embleton organised the prize-giving while Marion took on the reunion. It was held on a Saturday with the prize-giving in the morning followed by a Reunion Lunch. As this was a Golden Anniversary, Marion encouraged Margaret and Mary to invite various notables from the Society of Radiographers. The President, Alan Watson from Derby, Alexander (Sandy) Yule, Chairman

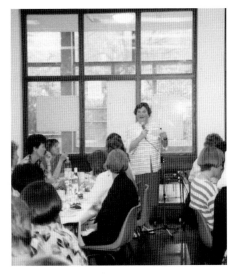

Image 91: A lunch to celebrate 50 years of radiography education at The Middlesex Hospital

178

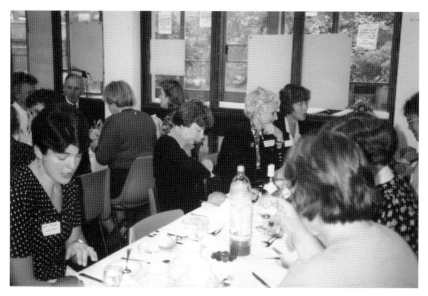

Image 92: The 50th anniversary lunch

of the Radiographers Board of the Council for Professions Supplementary to Medicine came from Cardiff, Michael Jordan, Society of Radiographers General Secretary (he would now be called Chief Executive) and Veronica Atherton, Education Officer for the College of Radiographers, both came from Kent. For all of them it was a considerable journey. On a Saturday morning in the lecture theatre of the medical school, with the platform party wearing golden roses in their buttonholes, that year's qualifying students received their certificates. The guest speaker was Sir Brian Windeyer, former Director of the Meyerstein Institute of Radiotherapy and of the Radiotherapy School, and past Dean of the Medical School, until his retirement in 1969. In front of a packed audience the proceedings were introduced by Margaret Wells, a former student and Superintendent of the Radiotherapy Department from 1974 to 1983. Mary Craig, Theo Gibbs, a former student and current Superintendent of the Nuclear Medicine Department, Dr Graham Whiteside, a retired Consultant Radiologist and lecturer, Marion Frank, and Jean Harvey, the current Superintendent of the X-ray Department gave short presentations covering a decade in the history of the Schools. It was during the previous week that it had become obvious that Marion was not intending that the notables and students' guests should attend the reunion lunch. Some would be coming from a long distance and no doubt would

179

be hungry. We very hastily put on coffee and doughnuts and desperately tried to hide our embarrassment when the first part of the day was over and we all trooped into the reunion lunch and everyone else went home.

When Julia Lovell, Principal of the Nuclear Medicine and Medical Ultrasound School, left in June 1985, Mary Lovegrove (Phillips) assumed charge of the Ultrasound programme; Mary Embleton took over administrative responsibility for the Nuclear Medicine course and undertook that qualification so that she could take full responsibility for the programme. The Superintendent of the Nuclear Medicine Department oversaw the curriculum in the interim so that Nuclear Medicine education and training at the Schools was able to continue. The Ultrasound programme was similarly overseen when Mary Lovegrove left and Jennifer Edie was in training. There was a great deal of co-operation and good will from all the clinical departments. The moneys released by the loss of Julia Lovell were used to upgrade the deputy principal in the diagnostic school to that of Principal II and provide additional funding of half a post to the radiotherapy school, which was used initially to part-fund a dual qualified (diagnostic and therapy) student teacher.

We were honoured when, as a member of the Schools' staff, Olive Deaville, who had trained as a teacher at Luton and Dunstable, and had previously spent time in the Schools gaining experience in a larger school as part of her teacher training, became President of the Society of Radiographers in July 1987, a role that had previously been held by both Mary Craig and Marion Frank.

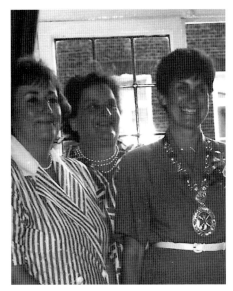

The HDCR programme incorporated the new syllabuses involving research projects and a different style of examination. The

Image 93: Olive Deaville, President, with Margaret McClellan and Marion Frank

TDCR syllabus was very formal and needed a great deal of work to complete. The Schools took an active part in the Society of Radiographers London and Home Counties branch teachers' tutorials and TDCR preparation. There were many overseas colleagues following programmes at all levels and so for a few years the new Schools continued to flourish and evolve. Margaret McClellan became an examiner for the Diploma, Higher Diploma and Teacher's Diploma examinations of the College of Radiographers.

In 1980 the Health Authority had sold Marlborough Court where many of its students had lived happily over the years. Accommodation was found for students in Warwickshire House, part of UCH, and then at John Astor House on The Middlesex site. It was at this time that Marion Frank retired, and she and her twin sister bought a two-bedroom flat together at Heron Court in Lancaster Gate. Whilst Marion's twin, Ellen, and her family were to have the use of it, it was primarily Marion's home and a safe haven for all itinerant radiographers and their friends from all over the world needing accommodation in London. You never knew who you were going to meet there. Marion would host many dinner parties, usually aimed at getting the group of invitees to undertake some task – like writing this book. Time spent there was filled with laughter, good food and excellent company, so the guests always agreed to do whatever was asked.

During the 1980s there was a drive by the College of Radiographers to upgrade the pre-registration training programme to that of a degree, and the staff of the Schools of Radiography at The Middlesex were in discussion with those of colleges and universities in London to this end as well. This was an uphill task because of serious opposition within the Ministry of Health, but it was supported by the other professions supplementary to medicine and by nursing. For many years the struggle continued but by the end of the 1980s a nationwide rationalisation programme of radiography education was under way. It was decreed by Government that the business of the Health Service was health and not the education of its professional employees and all hospital-based vocational schools were to be closed. Suddenly, and at very short notice, contracts for the education of professionals were to be competed for by universities, and degree programmes were to be introduced. The 1990s were therefore a period of great upheaval for all those involved in the education and training of all health professionals that were not medical. When the radiography schools were finally closed by Government edict in 1991, those in charge of placing the new educational contracts were amazed that the schools in London had not appeared, in the main, to regard themselves as rivals. They had always been prepared to help each other out in periods of shortage of teaching staff or specialist lecturers. A number of committees had been formed in London to enable a large amount of joint working. They developed the London and Home Counties Teachers' Group, the Further Education Committee, the Association of Radiography Teachers, many working parties and joint student activities. All this would now change.

Dealing with nursing and the professions supplementary to medicine was just the beginning of a tidal wave of change to hit the NHS Training and Education sector. One thing that did start to suffer was that previous co-operation and collaboration between all the schools in London and the Home Counties as degree programmes developed and rivalry began to show itself. Where there had once been goodwill, now there was suspicion. Where there had once been co-operation, now there would be fierce rivalry.

In NETRHA there were Schools of Radiography at The Middlesex & UCH, St. Bartholomew's, the Royal Free and the Royal London Hospitals. All were centres of excellence, and all were London Teaching Hospitals. Just as The Middlesex and UCH had been combined so had The Royal Free and Royal Northern hospitals and The Royal London with St Bartholomew's and Southend. Now it was time to combine all of these Schools into one large institution on a new site. This finally happened in December 1989, although in radiotherapy the Schools had effectively merged the previous summer. Sally Waddington, a radiotherapy teacher, had moved on to take up a post in Bristol, leaving Mary Embleton as the only qualified radiotherapy teacher. The therapy school did not now meet the College of Radiographers' required staffing level of three teachers, so the students' lecture programme was combined with those at St Bartholomew's and The Royal London Hospitals. Judy Taylor from The Royal London was appointed co-ordinator for the Diploma of the College of Radiographers' programme and Mary Embleton co-ordinator of the Higher Diploma which continued at The Middlesex School. In July 1990 Mary Embleton left, and responsibility for the Radiotherapy Higher Diploma programme was transferred to Angela Emerson at St Bartholomew's. Pam Cherry, who had been a student teacher at St Bartholomew's, was employed by The Middlesex when she qualified as a teacher; she was managerially responsible to Margaret McClellan and professionally responsible to Judy Taylor. Thus the amalgamation of the radiotherapy section was completed.

It was almost another two years before the School in Doran House transferred to join all the others in Charterhouse Square near the Barbican in the City of London, with their undergraduate and postgraduate programmes validated by City University. The Schools of Radiography Education Committee met for the last time on 10 July 1991 and was officially dissolved, and the official date for 'vacating the premises' was set for 7 October (a post-meeting note suggests it may have actually taken place on 1 November).

Those who were in charge of the combination of all the schools had learnt from the expensive experience of North West Thames Regional Health Authority, who chose to close their schools with no guarantee of jobs for any of their staff. They all received notice for the end of August 1989. This was very expensive, as all staff over fifty had to be early-retired, so that even if they got a job as part of a new contract, they had to be paid their National Health Service (NHS) pensions and lump sums with enhanced years, and those under that age had to be declared redundant, again with significant payments. Most of these staff had worked in the NHS for many years. NETRHA transferred all staff still employed by it in 1991 to the new establishment at Charterhouse College. It meant that the new school was over-staffed but this was deemed the less expensive option. With the exception of the part-time secretary who retired, the remaining staff at the Schools transferred to the new establishment. But first there were three parties. The first was a private one for the remaining staff held at Hatfield House where we went to a Tudor Dining Experience, along with several hundred others. It was a most enjoyable evening and in true fashion we ate, drank and laughed a lot. The second was a typical Middlesex Schools' Christmas Lunch for all who had worked in the Schools of Radiography since 1980. This took place in December 1990 and thirty one people were catered for. Of course, the sterilizer was in use to cook the Christmas pudding, and the traditional Christmas meal was served.

The third event was a more formal occasion in the Board Room of The Middlesex Hospital. The higher echelons of the health authority were there – we did not even know their names by now as they had all changed again. Nice words were

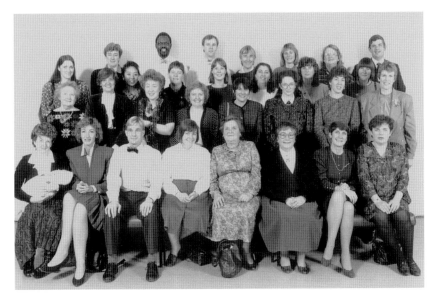

Image 94: The Christmas Lunch, December 1990

said about the Schools and what they had achieved over the years but, sadly, spoken by someone who had only just arrived and had no idea of the history that was being left behind. The best and most moving tribute came from the clinical staff. There was a gift for every teacher and it was given with warm words from a different member of staff each time. This was much appreciated by the teaching staff and a few tears were shed.

What happened to the Schools' building? During the latter part of the 1980s the School of Physiotherapy was informed by its Chartered Society that it did not meet the teaching accommodation requirements to support the number of students it had. There was no extra room available in Arthur Stanley House where the School of Physiotherapy was housed (about 500 yards away in Tottenham Street), and the fourth floor of Doran House, which was by now not much used, was redeveloped for them at some cost. Their new teaching facilities were never used but they did conform to their new requirements: precious money spent and not sensibly used except to meet the letter of the law.

As the physical move of the school contents was under way it became apparent that as clinical education was to continue at The Middlesex and UCH, arrangements needed to be made for this. Changing rooms, offices, a common room and a teaching room would be needed. The third floor of Doran House, Foley Street was ideal with very little alteration required. Mo Clarke, who was by then Superintendent of the Meyerstein Institute of Radiotherapy at The Middlesex, decided to fight the corner for the Middlesex radiotherapy students. It seemed clear to Margaret McClellan that staff and students, both diagnostic and radiotherapeutic, would benefit from sharing the new arrangements on the third floor. Mo Clarke wanted them to be separate. On the morning that both women met on the third floor with Stephen Golding, the young administrator tasked with sorting this out, the fur flew. Stephen was later heard to comment "God preserve me from menopausal women"!

The shared arrangements on the third floor lasted a couple of years and when that too was finally taken over, the students and clinical lecturers were moved to accommodation in the old School of Nursing on the other side of Foley Street. Teaching of the Diploma of Radionuclide Imaging course, which was then being run by Peter Hogg, also took place here, before that too, transferred to Charterhouse College.

The Middlesex Hospital closed in 2005 and patients and staff were housed at the new University College London Hospital at 235 Euston Road. A magnificent wing is named The Middlesex. Doran House has been redeveloped to provide affordable housing and externally does not look much different. The Outpatient department on Cleveland Street in the basement of which the radiography students had changed, and which had been an eighteenth-century building and both a Georgian and Victorian workhouse, was about to be pulled down by the owners, University College Hospital, to enable the building of 140 flats. In March 2011 it was declared to be a Grade II listed building and still remains, boarded up. The Middlesex Hospital site was sold to developers and the hospital pulled down to make way for re-development of the site. Then the economy tumbled and the owners could no longer afford the planned development. The hospital chapel, as a listed building, and the façade of the Meyerstein wing, are all that remains to give testament to a once proud institution of medical and radiographic excellence.

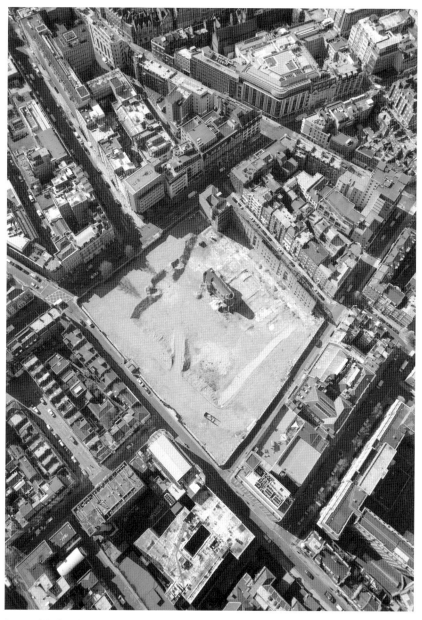

Image 95: Overhead view of The Middlesex Hospital's cleared site showing the Hospital Chapel and the Meyerstein façade still standing

BIBLIOGRAPHY

Chapter 1. Setting the Scene and the Hospital at War

Berry RJ. 'The radiologist as guinea pig: radiation hazards to man as demonstrated in early radiologists, and their patients'. *Journal of the Royal Society of Medicine*; vol 79, September 1986, pp.506-09.

Board of Governors' Minutes, *The Middlesex Hospital, (1933-1948)*. Archives of UCLH.

Bright J. *The Story of The Middlesex*. 1950, London, Adprint Ltd.

House booklets produced by the Middlesex Hospital.

Knox R. *Radiography, X-ray therapeutics and radium therapy*. 1915, London, A&C Black.

Miller AL. *The Middlesex – Two Hundred and Fifty Years 1745-1995*. 1995, printed and produced by the Middlesex Hospital.

Minutes of the House and Nursing Committees 1934-1943.

Minutes of the Nurse Education Committee 1944-1958.

Rawlinson Carole. *Middlesex Memories*. 2007. University College London Hospitals Charities, London

St George Saunders H. *The Middlesex Hospital 1745-1948*. 1949, London, Max Parrish and Co Ltd.

Chapter 2. Building a Modern Profession 1949 – 1979

Jordan M. *The Maturing Years - A History of The Society and College of Radiographers (1970-1995)*. 1995, The Society and College of Radiographers.

Minutes of the Schools of Radiography Education Committee (1947-1991).

Schools of Radiography (Diagnosis and Therapy), Golden Jubilee (1935-85), May 18th 1985.

Minutes of the Marlborough Court Committee 1949-1953.

Personal letter from Graham Buckley, Administrator, The Middlesex Hospital, April 2010 re Marlborough Court.

Syllabus for the Diploma of the Society of Radiographers, The Society of Radiographers, 1976, The Society of Radiographers.

Syllabus for the Membership of the Society of Radiographers Examination, 1960, The Society of Radiographers, London.

Chapter 3. Technical Innovation 1895 – 1991

Eastwood WS. 'The design of Caesium Sources for Teletherapy'. *British Journal of Radiology,* 1960.

Grigg ERN. *The Trail of the Invisible Light.* 1965, Illinois, Charles C Thomas.

Gupta VK. 1995. 'Brachytherapy – past, present and future'. *Journal of Medical Physics*; **20**: 31–38.

Donald I. 'Investigation of Abdominal Masses by Pulsed Ultrasound', *Lancet,* 1958, 7 June.

Kurjak A (Jun. 2000). 'Ultrasound scanning - Prof. Ian Donald (1910-1987)'. *Eur. J. Obstet. Gynecol. Reprod. Biol.* (IRELAND); **90** (2): 187–189.

Mould R. *A century of X-rays and Radioactivity in Medicine.* 1993, Institute of Physics, London.

Stewart, Alice M, Webb JW, Giles BD, Hewitt D. 1956. 'Preliminary Communication: Malignant Disease in Childhood and Diagnostic Irradiation In-Utero,' *Lancet,* 1956; **2**: 447.

Treatment Machines for External Beam Radiotherapy. See link to web site: http://www-naweb.iaea.org/nahu/dmrp/pdf_files/Chapter5.pdf.

Windeyer, Sir Brian (Obituary). *BMJ*, vol 309, 1994 Nov 19, p.1367.

Williams ES, Ell PJ. *The Institute of Nuclear Medicine – The First 25 Years*. 1986, London, CW Printing, Sevenoaks, Kent.

Chapter 4. Reaching Out

McClellan M. Report of a Questionnaire addressed to a small number of qualified radiographers on the influence and success of the post qualification courses and experience offered at the Schools of Radiography, The Middlesex Hospital 2009 (unpublished).

Minutes of the Schools of Radiography Education Committee (1947-1991).

Chapter 5. Mary and Marion

Lucy Mary Craig

Radiography, December 1957, Vol. XXIII, No. 276.

Radiography, February 1975, Vol. XLI, No. 482.

Marion Frank

'History of ISSRT' on ISSRT website

Personal communication and interviews with Marion Frank.

Windeyer, Sir Brian (Obituary). *BMJ*; **309**, 1994 Nov 19, p.1367

Jordan, M, Obituary of Marion Frank. *Synergy News*, 2011, Oct, p.6.

Leaflet issued at the unveiling of a monument to 3 Troop 10 (IA) Commando -The Story behind the Monument at Penhelyg Park, Aberdyfi.

Chapter 6. Memories

Personal memories.

Minutes of the Nurse Education Committee (1944-1965).

Minutes of the Radiography and Radiotherapy Education and Welfare Committee (1965-1991).

Chapter 7. The Merger and the End

Minutes of the Radiography and Radiotherapy Education and Welfare Committee (1965-1991).

Syllabus and Regulations for the Diploma of The College of Radiographers and for the Higher Diploma of The College of Radiographers, 1982, 1988 revision, The College of Radiographers.

Schools of Radiography (Diagnosis and Therapy), Golden Jubilee (1935-85), May 18th 1985.

APPENDIX A

Middlesex Schools of Radiography lists of subjects and time allocation

1935-1945 (18 months)	1946 (2 years)
Requirement for entry School leaving certificate, later withdrawn.	**Requirement for entry** School leaving certificate, certificates in First Aid and Home Nursing
General physics, x-ray physics, radioactivity (Physicist)	**Basic Physics, electricity & magnetism** (Prof Roberts, Dr Cooke) 62 hours
First Aid & Radiation Protection (Radiologist)	
Anatomy and Physiology (Radiologist)	**Anatomy** (Dr Graham Hodgson) 34 hours
Electricity and Apparatus Construction (Morgan Davies)	**Apparatus Construction** (Morgan Davies) 48 hours
Photography (Photographer)	**Photography** (Sister Parbery) 12 hrs +2 weeks @ Kodak
Practical Radiography	**Radiographic Technique** (Radiologist) 24 hours
Radiation Therapy, Radium, Ultra violet radiation (Sister Bristow)	**Radiotherapy** (Dr Shorvon & Sister Craig) 36 hours
General discipline and organisation of students (resident radiographer)	**Radiography and radiotherapy revision** (Radiologist and radiotherapist) 16 hours

Subjects and time allocation from Society/College of Radiographers syllabi

Part 1 subjects

Society of Radiographers Syllabus 1960 (2 years)	Society of Radiographers Syllabus 1976 (2 years)	College of Radiographers Syllabus 1982 (rev.1988) (3 years)
Requirement for entry 4 or 5 GCE O' Levels depending on subject or equivalent	**Requirement for entry** 4 or 5 GCE O' Levels depending on subject or equivalent	**Requirement for entry** 7 GCSE passes: 5 O' Level grade C or above, 2 A' Level Grade D (or equivalent to 4 points)
Physics *Suggested* number of lectures 50 hours *plus* tutorials and practical demonstrations	**Physics** *Suggested* number of lectures:100 hours *including* tutorials and practical demonstrations	**Physics** *Minimum* number of teaching hours: 150 hours *including* tutorials and practical demonstrations
Hospital Practice and Care of the Patient 15 hours plus tutorials and demonstrations	**Hospital Practice and Care of the Patient** 60 hours	**Hospital Practice and Care of the Patient** 70 hours
Anatomy and Physiology 60 hours plus tutorials	**Anatomy and Physiology** 120 hours	**Anatomy and Physiology** 150 hours

Part 2 subjects

Society of Radiographers Syllabus 1960 (2 years)	Society of Radiographers Syllabus 1976 (2 years)	College of Radiographers Syllabus 1982 (rev.1988) (3 years)
Equipment for Diagnostic Radiography 30 hours plus tutorials	**Equipment for Diagnostic Radiography** 80 hours	**Equipment for Diagnostic Radiography** 100 hours
Radiographic Photography 30 hours plus tutorial	**Radiographic Photography** 60 hours	**Radiographic Photography** 90 hours
Radiographic Technique 80 – 100 hours plus tutorials	**Radiographic Technique** 160 – 200 hours	**Radiographic Technique** 300 hours
Radiotherapy Physics and Equipment 30 hours plus tutorials	**Radiotherapy Physics and Equipment** 60 hours	**Radiotherapy Physics and Equipment** 100 hours
Radiotherapy Technique 60 hours plus tutorials	**Radiotherapy Technique** 150 hours	**Radiotherapy Technique** 150 hours
	Principles of Radiotherapy and Oncology 90 hours	**Principles of Radiotherapy and Oncology** 90 hours

APPENDIX B

The Role of the Professional Body and Statutory Regulatory Body and the qualifications they awarded or recognised

The Society and College of Radiographers

The Society of Radiographers, and later its subsidiary the College of Radiographers, as the professional body for Radiographers, was from 1921 until the early 1990s the examination and awarding body for all professional qualifications for Radiographers. In 1931 the education subcommittee of the Society advised that it was best for teaching to take place at centres recognised by the Society. The first school inspection took place in 1932 when the first four schools were visited and recognised by the Society as training centres.

By the end of the 1960s there was concern that not everyone passing the Membership of the Society of Radiographers (MSR) examination joined the professional body. It was therefore decided that the examination should become the Diploma of the Society of Radiographers (DSR). The qualification was noted as being in Diagnostic Radiography (R) or Radiotherapy (T).

During the 1970s the Society took on an increasing role in industrial relations and restructuring took place, with the formation of the College of Radiographers as part of the organisation.

The Society of Radiographers is a membership organisation, which is the professional, educational and trade union body for radiographers and other clinical staff working in the field of radiography.

The College of Radiographers is the charitable subsidiary of the Society. Its objectives are directed towards education, research and activities that support the practice of radiography and allied disciplines.

As the setting and examining of curricula, the awarding of qualifications and the setting of standards for, and inspection of training centres where all education activities took place came under the role of the College of Radiographers, the qualification became the Diploma of the College of Radiographers (DCR).

The Society and College of Radiographers also set the syllabus, and was the examination authority and awarding body for a number of further qualifications for radiographers, which are listed below:

The Fellowship of the Society of Radiographers (FSR), was introduced in 1945/6 and was later replaced by the Higher Diploma of the Society of Radiographers (HDSR), and finally became the Higher Diploma of the College of Radiographers (HDCR). The Fellowship became an honorary award conferred in recognition of service to the profession.

The first recognition for teachers was the Teacher's Endorsement (I Ė), introduced in the mid-1950s for those already holding the FSR. In 1968 this was replaced with the Teacher's Diploma of the Society of Radiographers (TDSR), which later became the Teacher's Diploma of the College (TDCR). Candidates for the Teacher's Diploma were required to hold the HDSR/HDCR and the City and Guilds Further Education Teacher's Certificate (FETC).

The other qualifications of the College of Radiographers for radiographers specialising in specific areas of practice were:

i. The Diploma in Nuclear Medicine (DNM), which later became the Diploma in Radionuclide Imaging (DRI).
ii. The Diploma in Medical Ultrasound (DMU).
iii. The Management Diploma of the College of Radiographers (MDCR).

Between 1973 and 1994 the Society/College of Radiographers sent 426 notices giving notification to Training Centres of information and requirements. These were known as TC documents and were identified by number.

The Statutory Regulatory Body: The Radiographers Board at The Council for Professions Supplementary to Medicine (CPSM)

The CPSM was a statutory regulatory body set up to implement the PSM 1960 Act. Its role was to supervise the activities of the Boards established for each of the health professions that the CPSM regulated.

The main role of the Radiographers Board was to protect the public by maintaining a register of those who were fit to practise. In order to practise in the National Health Service radiographers were required to register with the Radiographers Board at the CPSM. The qualifications and experience of overseas radiographers were assessed by the Board to ascertain whether they were fit to practise in the United Kingdom.

When the Society and College of Radiographers revised the syllabus for the MSR/DSR/DCR examination, it had to be submitted to the Radiographers' Board for approval and via the Board to Privy Council for confirmation of approval. The Board also approved institutions that trained radiographers and visited Schools of Radiography to ensure their suitability. This role did not extend to the further qualifications taken by radiographers following qualification.

The Council for Professions Supplementary to Medicine (CPSM) was later replaced by the Health Professions Council (HPC).

Summary of Society and College of Radiographers' educational awards

		Awarded
Qualification examination		
MSR	Membership of the Society of Radiographers	1921 – 1970
DSR	Diploma of the Society of Radiographers	1971 – 1976
DCR	Diploma of the College of Radiographers	1977 – 1996
Post Diploma Qualifications		
FSR	Fellowship of the Society of Radiographers	1949 - 1967
HDSR	Higher Diploma of the Society of Radiographers	1968 - 1976
HDCR	Higher Diploma of the College of Radiographers	1977 - 1996
TE	Teacher's Endorsement	1956 - 1967
TDSR	Teacher's Diploma of the Society of Radiographers	1967 - 1976
TDCR	Teacher's Diploma of the College of Radiographers	1977 – 1993
DNM	Diploma in Nuclear Medicine	1973 – 1982
DRI	Diploma in Radionuclide Imaging	1982 – 1995
DMU	Diploma in Medical Ultrasound	1977 – 1997
MDCR	Management Diploma of College of Radiographers	1984 - 1993

APPENDIX C

Countries from which students came to study at The Middlesex Hospital

Australia	Israel	Seychelles
Barbados	Italy	Sierra Leone
Botswana	Japan	Singapore
Canada	Jamaica	South Africa
Cyprus	Jordan	South Yemen
Denmark	Kenya	Sri Lanka
Ethiopia	Kuwait	Syria
Fiji	Lebanon	Somalia
Finland	Libya	Switzerland
Ghana	Malta	Thailand
Gibraltar	Malaysia	Trinidad
Hong Kong	Mauritius	Uganda
Holland	Mexico	United Kingdom
India	New Zealand	United States of America
Indonesia	Nigeria	Zambia
Iran	Norway	Zimbabwe
Iraq	Poland	
Ireland	Qatar	(52)

APPENDIX D

Principals and Directors of the Schools of Radiography

School of Diagnostic Radiography Principals

1935 – 1949	Sister Joan Parbery
1949 – 1981	Miss Marion Frank
1981 – 1991	Miss Margaret McClellan

School of Diagnostic Radiography Directors*

1935 – 1955	Sir Harold Graham Hodgson
1955 – 1966	Dr Frederick Campbell Golding
1966 – 1980	Dr J Norman Pattinson
1980 – 1984	Dr Maurice Raphael

School of Therapy Radiography Principals

1935 – 1942	Sister RM Smith
1942 – 1974	Sister L Mary Craig
1974 – 1980	Miss Anne Wells
1980 – 1990	Mrs Mary Embleton

School of Therapy Radiography Directors

1935 – 1969	Professor Sir Brian Windeyer
1969 – 1979	Miss Margaret Snelling
1979 – 1984*	Professor Roger Berry

School of Nuclear Medicine and Medical Ultrasound**

1975 – 1977	Mrs Marilyn Swann (Walton)
1980 – 1985	Miss Julia Lovell

School of Nuclear Medicine and Medical Ultrasound

1975 – 1985	Professor Edward Williams

Chairmen of the Schools Education Committee
1980 – 1988   Professor Roger Berry
1988 – 1991   Dr Maurice Raphael

*Directors of the Schools. In 1984 following the amalgamation with University College Hospital the directors' roles were divided between the Chairman of the Education Committee and the consultants representing each discipline

**Although no Principal specific to Nuclear Medicine and Ultrasound was appointed after 1985, these specialist courses continued under the responsibility of The Middlesex Schools

APPENDIX E

Middlesex staff/former students elected President of Society of Radiographers

1957 – 1958   Miss L. Mary Craig
                      Radiotherapy Principal

1967 – 1968   Miss Marion Frank
                      Diagnostic Principal

1973 – 1974   Miss A. Nanette Plowman
                      Former radiotherapy student and Superintendent at UCH

1982 – 1983   Miss Christine Soutter
                      Former Student (D & T) and Radiotherapy teacher (T)

1987 – 1988   Mrs Olive Deaville
                      Deputy Principal, Diagnostic

1996 – 1997   Mrs Julia Henderson
                      Former student (D & T) and student teacher (D)

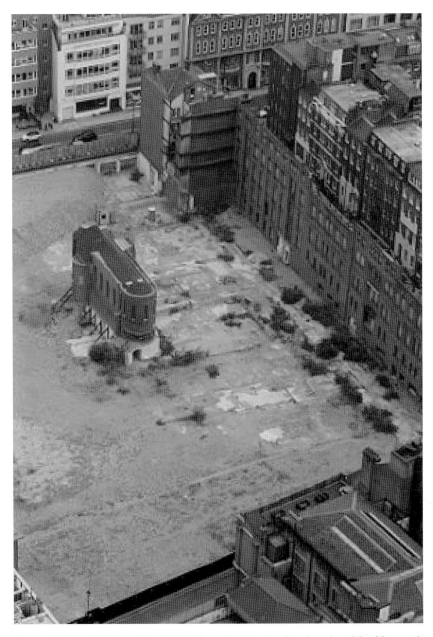

Image 96: The Middlesex Hospital building site, showing the chapel and the Meyerstein façade still standing

Further copies of this book can be obtained by contacting Patricia Ducker p.ducker.barber@btinternet.com